Jack and Jill Spratt's Amazing Journey to Healthful Eating

by

Sam Biondo, ScD

An Explorer's Guide to Delicious Plant Based Diet Styles

Text copyright © 2015 Sam Biondo
All Rights Reserved

Cover Illustrated by William Nelson

Conflict of Interest Statement

The author and publisher of this book declare that there are no conflicts of interest. There are no financial interests in or arrangements with any company whose product was used in this book or is referred to in this book or any other situations that may have potentially biased this book, its conclusions, implications, or opinion statements. These include direct or indirect sources of funding for the author and publisher. In addition, there are no personal relationships or arrangements with any individuals or organizations discussed in this book or referred to in this book or any other situations that may have potentially biased this book, its conclusions, implications, or opinion statements.

Disclaimer of Endorsements

Reference in this book to any specific commercial products, services, or links to Web sites, or the use of any firm, or corporation name is for the information of readers and does not constitute endorsement.

*Dedicated to
my Children*

Contents

Preface	3
Chapter One: Resolutions	9
Chapter Two: Weights and Measures	19
Chapter Three: Food Labels	42
Chapter Four: Don't Eat *That!*	48
Chapter Five: Eat This	71
Chapter Six: Tools and Aids	98
Chapter Seven: Filling Your Shopping Cart and Stocking Your Pantry	105
Chapter Eight: Dining at Restaurants & Dining with Friends and Relatives	117
Chapter Nine: Plan Ahead and Be Prepared	123
Chapter Ten: Satisfying Your Appetite for Knowledge	139
Appendix	146
References	150

Preface

Jack Spratt ate healthful fats, his wife ate greens and beans. They had a propensity for high nutrient density. Read this book to learn what that means.

The whimsical cover belies the serious topics that are discussed in this book. This book is about escaping the clutches of the Standard American Diet (SAD) to promote health and reduce chronic disease risk through the consumption of healthful diets. Trying to achieve that goal can seem like piloting a dinghy on an ocean voyage. Perhaps fittingly the journey is over water, the life giving liquid and essential nutrient.

This explorer's guide will help you navigate a journey to a healthful, high quality lifestyle focused on eating delicious foods that are best for you, while halting your unhealthy eating habits, and arresting the desire for popular, irresistible unhealthful foods. Regardless of whether your motivation is an aspiration for healthy living, a desire to lose weight, concerns about the ethics of eating animal product, or some combination of those reasons and possibly others, this book will guide your journey to a healthful, toothsome destination.

We strived to make reading this book easy and informative, and hopefully an interesting and pleasant experience. But we can't promise your journey will be always smooth and uneventful. A lot will depend on you. You will be the captain of your ship, steering the course with a pioneering spirit. Like an ocean voyage to a distant land, there are many paths that you can take, and upon arrival there will be entire new worlds to explore. Many have made the passage to healthy eating and many more people are continuing to do so. Most of them had to sail unchartered waters. When they disembarked they discovered varied and changing landscapes, and new horizons that brightened their lives.

Unfortunately, many other voyagers, particularly those struggling to lose weight, have fallen off the wagon and failed to achieve their goals. That is not surprising since it is well known that most dieters can't maintain their target weights. We frequently hear the complaint, *"I tried eating plant based, processed food products but it was like eating cardboard."* Or, *"I just don't have time to shop for stuff that is hard to find and learn how to cook it too."*

Sincere dieters who tried really hard but had bad experiences might be able to get back on course with some guidance, better eating choices, and perseverance. Skeptics who really don't want to give up addicting junk food and unhealthful dietary behaviors may unknowingly be treading a path leading to chronic diseases. Those chronic diseases can include type 2 diabetes, cardiovascular disease, and cardiovascular risk factors (high blood cholesterol and triglyceride, high blood pressure, etc.), respiratory diseases such as asthma, musculoskeletal disorders such as osteoarthritis and low back pain, several cancers, and depression[1]. Additionally excessive body fat causes other metabolic pathologies, such as non-alcoholic fatty liver disease, and unhealthful dietary behavior is also associated with an increased incidence of chronic kidney disease[2].

You may have to face formidable challenges. You will have to navigate a maze of contradictory, confusing information and misinformation, including controversial government food "policy" documents[3], in your efforts to discover which healthful food is best for you. You may also encounter difficulties finding some of the foods and products you are seeking. It is likely you will have to confront food addiction and preferences for unhealthful foods, resist the temptations of seductive advertising, and the enticement of convenient, ready available, delicious, unhealthful foods. But the experience and knowledge will enable you to make smarter and wiser dietary choices. And perhaps surprisingly, your individual sense of what food is "delicious" will gradually change.

There are no fixed GPS solutions for your voyage. This guide does not dictate menus or recipes to follow the first days, or weeks, nor does it attempt to prescribe specific foods you must eat because we all have different individual flavor preferences. Nearly every person's sense of flavor is subtly different.
Your personal taste and cultural traditions need to dictate your dietary choices. There is no single best diet. Your diet will have to be tailored to best suit your needs from a myriad of different options available to you among the various sources of healthful foods.

This guide will empower you with the knowledge that you need to make informed decisions about what you eat, and it includes many suggestions that will help you select among healthful options. The aim is to help smooth your journey through the choppy seas and make the transition to healthful eating pleasant and productive.

> Note regarding the use in this book of the words **"healthful"** and **"healthy:"**
>
> Healthful is the correct word to describe something that promotes good health.
>
> Healthy describes something (plants, people and other animals) in good health. However, due to the widespread usage of healthy in place of healthful to describe foods and diets, the words healthy and healthful are used as synonyms.

Countless healthful food options are available to you. Consider an elementary example concerning the variety of different salad combinations you could create from these ingredients: If your dinner salad is comprised of green vegetables (kale, arugula, watercress, spinach, etc.), berries (blueberries, strawberries, blackberries, grapes, etc.), seeds (pumpkin seeds, hemp seeds, chia seeds, sunflower seeds, etc.), and vegetables (carrots, onions, bell peppers, mushrooms, etc.), you could easily create different salads every day for nearly five years with products purchased from your grocery stores. Of course there are many more options for each of those four food categories and many more food categories, and therefore exponentially more combinations of different salad selections. Also keep in mind that you are in the driver's seat, choosing the best tasting foods from among the innumerable healthy food options that are available to you.

The benefits that you achieve will be determined by the goals you set and the efforts you make to achieve them. There will be different risks and rewards associated with each of the major diets.

> **"Diet"** is frequently the term used to describe a dietary regimen for losing weight, but in this book the word diet means all of the food we eat in a particular time period-daily, weekly, monthly, etc. or lifestyles alternatives that your choose.

The major diets or dietary lifestyles are safe passage routes for your journey to healthy eating. Granted it is difficult to choose a healthful diet style because there is so much conflicting information available today in magazines, books, TV, and the Internet. However, there is a growing body of scientific evidence and clinical experience that support diets with lots of fruits, vegetables, and whole grains, along with healthy sources of protein and fats. And there is a well established set of the major healthful diets or diet style alternatives including for example:

A **nutritarian** diet style focused on healthful, nutrient dense foods that are most favorable to long-term survival[4].

A **vegan** diet style based on the support of animal rights or other altruistic reasons that doesn't permit the consumption of animals or animal products.

Vegetarian diet styles that can include the consumption of dairy products and eggs.

A **flexitarian** diet style that is vegetarian but occasionally includes meat and fish[5].

Each of those plant based diet style options can improve your quality of life, reduce the risks of diseases and disability, and help you to live a longer, fuller, happy life. There are certainly many other plant-based diet and diet style options that are healthful but most of them are not as credible and well documented. This book will provide useful guidance to adopting them as well.

This is a journey of discovery that can be enormously beneficial. It can be inspirational and exciting, but it will likely require great resolve and perseverance. The journey may not be easy but it will be well worth the effort.

We strived to make the information in this book clear and easy to follow. We tried to avoid the oversimplification of complex mechanisms and over complication of simple issues. And it was not always wise to ignore relevant but inconsequential information because there is often value in knowing what things you don't have to know and why you can ignore them. For example, in the chapter titled Weights and Measures, you will learn why you can ignore the many measures and commercial devices to estimate body fat and body mass index.

Also don't be alarmed to see math formulas in this book. Some will inform you about things you may have heard about that are not really useful. Others may satisfy your curiosity or demystify jargon, and some math equations may be useful to other people but you won't need to learn to use them. Again, there is value in knowing what you can ignore. On the other hand, it is not a good idea to ignore the information on food product labels, but once you know which additives to avoid you won't have to devote anymore time trying to decipher deceptive information on labels for unhealthful products.

Many advocates ignore or understate the challenges of converting from a Western-style to a plant based diet style. Among them are the obstacles created by the social aspects of food and eating, and the hurdles engendered by our habitats – where we live, work, and play. We live in obesity promoting (obesogenic) environments where food is in abundance and societal trends encourage patterns of overeating and little physical activity[6]. The vast majority of our population does not grow their own fruits and vegetables, or live and work near vegan and vegetarian grocery stores and restaurants. Shopping times and distances can easily double, triple or quadruple in the quest for healthful foods and meals.

At an individual level most people do not invest a huge amount of time thinking about their diets. And they are not willing to give up the satisfaction of comfort foods – food prepared in a simple or traditional way that reminds them of home, family, or friends. They are foods that people eat to make them feel better. In fact people can be driven towards comfort foods even when they are not really hungry. To some people eating familiar foods can be viewed as the best, most important part of a person's day. Giving up comfort foods completely is emotionally difficult.

Exposure to conflicting news about the health benefits of foods, vitamins and supplements creates confusion and backlash against nutrition recommendations, making many people –particularly those addicted to comfort foods – more likely to ignore not only the contradictory information, but also widely accepted nutritional advice. Confronted by a never ending stream of dietary *villains du jour* – such as butter and sugar – and with the knowledge that some of the old villains have been exonerated and have humbled their nemeses – namely margarine (without trans fat) and artificial sweeteners – even the most authoritative nutritional pronouncements of dreadful risks and life saving benefits can create skepticism or confusion that tends to fall on deaf ears. It's enough to want to make even sainted sailors resort to salty language. *"Tell it to the marines,"* the scoffers say. This book will help you ignore the skeptics, stay the course, and ride the crests of the waves on a journey to healthful eating.

This is a factual guide-book, not an encyclopedia. It does not provide an exhaustive listing of foods, spices, or dos and don'ts. We do not endorse any food products. And while recipes are not included, we encourage the readers to forage for pleasing recipes among the many tens of thousands that are readily available. Our aim is to provide enough detail to enable you to direct your own diet style change so you can discover the benefits of healthful eating.

The First five chapters contain some thought provoking questions in sections titled "Food for Thought."

In Chapter One, "Resolutions," the popular reasons for considering plant based diets are briefly reviewed. Important health benefits of plant based diets are identified. Health impacts of poor diet choices are discussed. The nutritional sciences studies dilemma that creates public confusion and skeptical consumers is examined. And barriers that must be addressed for the successful transition to healthful eating are explained. Some leading plant based diet styles are previewed.

In Chapter Two, "Weights and Measures," methods for estimating healthy weight and body fat are critically examined and their usage, validity and potential value for individual users is discussed. A procedure to monitor weight is suggested. Information is presented on the molecular nature of digestion, appetite, and energy metabolism. Diet formulation, nutrient density, and various attempts to apply the nutrient density concept to profile or rate foods are reviewed.

Chapter Three, "Labels," is concerned with seeking accurate information from credible sources concerning the nutrient and energy content of food products. You will discover that FDA and USDA regulations for food product labels are important to inform our knowledge of nutritional contents and production methods, but food labels do not provide a sufficient list of nutrients for a comprehensive analysis. And there are many regulatory loopholes that cause concerns.

Chapter Four is titled "Don't Eat That!" This chapter furnishes guidance on avoiding or limiting harmful substances in foods, food products, additives, and nutritional supplements. Trans fats, saturated fats and carbohydrates with high glycemic foods are discussed. The risks associated with the excessive consumption of vitamins or minerals are presented. The health issues with processed meat and sodium are identified. Aids are suggested for informing decisions on supplements. The federal regulations and the health risks of supplements and food additives are reviewed and the most controversial additives are discussed. Guidance is provided on consumption practices.

Chapter Five, "Eat This!" address the question, *"What foods are healthful foods?"* This chapter identifies the key attributes of healthful foods and the legal definitions for references to healthful food products. It discusses published government guidelines for planning and assessing healthy diets. The nourishing characteristics of healthful foods are identified. Suggestions are presented on ways to enhance the flavor of boring or objectionable foods and create savory and delicious meals without compromising nutritional values. Healthful plant based meat substitutes and vegan protein sources that can provide new and familiar savory textures and flavors are profiled. Information is presented concerning the relationship of fruit and vegetable consumption with wellness and the development of chronic disease.

There are several well known food pyramids that are supposed to suggests the types and frequencies of foods that should be enjoyed for health. Chapter Five identifies the common food groups in healthy plant based diets and discuss the considerable differences in their importance and range of servings for each of the food groups in nine well known food pyramids. Readers are encouraged to construct their own food pyramids, which can be used for purchasing produce and food products and planning meals. A detailed example, which we named *The Toothsome Triangle* pyramid, is presented.

Chapter Six, "Tools and Aids," provides guidance and focuses on devices to facilitate your transition to a healthful plant based diet. It recaps some of the key take-aways of previous chapters, furnishes additional suggestions, and identifies a few useful devices that you might want to add to your shopping list.

Chapter Seven, "Filling Your Shopping Cart and Stocking Your Pantry," demonstrates how food pyramids can be used to help construct shopping lists for staples to store in your refrigerator, freezer, and pantry. This concept is illustrated in a detailed example using the Toothsome Triangle from Chapter Four to formulate a hypothetical shopping list. Some grocery shopping tips and food preparations suggestions are included. Time and cost tradeoffs are also discussed.

Chapter Eight, "Dining at Restaurants & Dining with Friends or Relatives," contains tips and suggestions for making healthful food choices and strategies to employ to avoid unhealthful food when dining at restaurants, with friends or with relatives.

Chapter Nine, "Plan Ahead and Be Prepared," includes guidance and discussions of several important topics including: Ensuring access to healthful foods throughout the day; seeking foods that taste good; informing your doctor about your diet style; changing taste preferences; building and maintaining a healthful food inventory; the pace of your transition to healthful eating; controlling cravings; diet and sleep tradeoffs; inverting the food pyramid; cooking issues and tips; what to do about dessert; weight and exercise; and peer-base social support. And it also contains a number of incisive questions to ask about food and health claims and announcements to help you determine their credibility and how important the results are for you personally.

Chapter Ten," Satisfying Your Appetite for Knowledge," provides numerous links to the electronic version of articles and books on topics that might be of interest to the readers.

The Appendix contains a list of phytochemicals included in the aggregate nutrient density index (ANDI) scoring and a table of ethylene production and sensitivity of perishable fruits and vegetables. Finally, the endnotes are contained in the References.

Chapter One: Resolutions

"Resolve to perform what you ought; perform without fail what you resolve." - Benjamin Franklin

There are many different reasons for people to adopt a plant based diet that is focused on eating healthful foods: Some people are influenced by magazine articles and books, or by watching health-and-lifestyle TV shows. They can be fans inspired by news about vegan or vegetarian celebrities. Or co-opted friends or relatives of vegans, or vegetarians. Others are not happy with the way they look – perhaps a bit broad in the beam – and want to lose weight, even though they are not obese. And they may be among the numerous altruistic people (over a million vegans in the U.S. in 2008) driven by compassion for animals and the desire to champion animal rights[7].

Additionally, many people are concerned about the significant health risks (e.g. hypertension, obesity) of poor nutrition, especially those who have been diagnosed with nutrition related diseases (e.g. heart disease, stroke, type 2 diabetes, cancer, osteoarthritis). Regardless of the reasons, everyone who invests the effort to transition to a healthier diet can expect to experience an enhanced quality of life and other significant benefits from eating healthful foods.

Health Impacts of Diet

Considerable knowledge concerning the profound impacts of our diets has established which foods are regarded as "healthful foods." They are foods that provide our essential nutrients, plus energy to sustain growth, health, and life while satiating hunger and reducing the risk of certain disease such as stroke, obesity, cancer, or diabetes. It is widely reported that healthful foods can also reverse certain diseases or disabilities, protect against dementia, increase life expectancy, help you lose excess weight, reduce medical expenses, and provide many other benefits that are identified below.

By contrast, it is well know that "unhealthful foods" are linked to stroke, obesity, cancer, diabetes, dementia, other diseases and disabilities, diminishing the quality of life, reducing life expectancy, adding excess body weight, increasing medical expenses, and creating many other harmful occurrences and losses. Accordingly, rational people should elect to choose healthy, nutritious foods and avoid unhealthy, nutrient-poor foods – especially *"junk foods"* – even though they are palatable, convenient, and inexpensive. Junk foods are high calorie foods, i.e., <u>energy-dense</u>, with little or no nutrients.

Of course, the amount of food you eat is very important. Eating too much of any food or too little of the essential nutrients can be harmful. And regardless of their nutrient and energy contents it is wise to always avoid foods that contain harmful ingredients.

By definition so-called <u>nutrient dense</u> foods provide the greatest amount of nutrients for the fewest calories. The concept of nutrient density has become well established during the past decade. There are several systems for judging nutrient density. Basically, the nutrient density of a substance is described by a ratio of the nutrient content (numerator) per (or divided by) its energy content (denominator). The energy content is stated in calories. Choosing nutrient dense plant based foods, like vegetables and fruits, over energy-dense foods will allow you to obtain many of the benefits of healthful foods.

Lower blood pressure, lower cholesterol, lower blood sugar, lower rates of cancer, and healthy weight loss, are some of the benefits that have been linked to plant-based diets. Dramatically decreased occurrences of cancer, heart disease, and strokes, with concomitant increase in life expectancy have been reported in numerous studies.

In contrast, diets characterized by a significant share of highly processed and refined foods and high content of sugars, salt, fat and protein from red meat, contribute to the development of metabolic disorders and the obesity epidemic. Excessive body fat causes metabolic pathologies, such as insulin resistance, type 2 diabetes, abnormally high blood lipids, cardiovascular diseases, hypertension, non-alcoholic fatty liver disease and cancer. The combination of nutrients typical for those diets contributes to chronic kidney disease. Additionally, such diets are associated with a chronic inflammatory process that is involved in all stages of atherosclerosis development and is increasingly recognized as a universal mechanism of various chronic degenerative diseases, such as autoimmune diseases, some neoplasms or osteoporosis[8].

According to Dr. Joel Fuhrman the author of the nutritarian diet, which features the consumption of the most micronutrient-rich foods, *"The deadly combination of processed wheat, processed foods, and too much animal products are scientifically shown to lead to weight gain, diabetes, heart disease, cancer, premature aging, and dementia."*[9]

Nutritional Sciences Dilemma

The profound health impacts of diet should come as no surprise to the reader, but it is also not surprising that many people are seemingly not aware or ignore the need for diet style changes that are driven by well publicized advances in nutritional science. Nutritional science is controversial.

There is an historical, widespread lack of respect for nutritional science that is well earned. Numerous instances of food and health reports with news of contradictory nutritional findings, such as the one hundred year battle of butter versus margarine, have spawned generations of health conscious consumers and many nutritional science skeptics[10].

The traditional controversial nature of nutrition science has undermined the public's confidence and contributed to confusion and skepticism. Surveys have shown that the majority of people believed experts would in the next few years completely change their recommendations about which foods were healthy and which were not. The skeptics' predictions have often come true. Frequently cited examples include red meat, eggs, salt, margarine, avocados, coffee, and whole milk.

And the confusion goes on: There was once widespread belief of a clear link between fiber and colon cancer, but subsequently stronger evidence found that fiber intake has no direct link with colon cancer[11]. Nevertheless, it is widely accepted that dietary fiber is a necessary component of a healthy diet and is required for normal bowel movement. However, a study published in 2012 claims to have confirmed that the previous strongly-held belief that dietary fiber helps constipation is but a myth. The authors reported that contrary to popularly held beliefs, reducing or stopping dietary fiber intake improves constipation and its associated symptoms[12].

Turning from dietary fiber to dietary fat, a recent study that questioned whether fats from fish or vegetable oils are healthier than those in meat or butter is another good example of the kind of information that can create confusion[13].

The failure to convincingly address the controversial and unresolved nature of the reported associations between dietary factors and disease processes has become a distinguishing characteristic of nutrition science. There are many contributing factors, beginning with the research process. We will briefly discuss a few of them.

Nutritional research is plagued by reliance on **observational studies** due to the absence of **randomized clinical trial** (RTC) evidence for many diet-disease relations. The use of RTCs is limited by expense and logistical challenges. Yet nutritional science experts claim that observational studies, if well designed and conducted appropriately, can be a valuable and effective approach to determining associations between specific exposures and outcomes, and they are the method of choice when it is not possible to conduct randomized trials.

However, S. Stanley Young, former director of bioinformatics at the National Institute of Statistical Sciences has presented evidence of a false discovery rate for observational studies of greater than ninety percent[14]. Dr. Young was recently quoted in the Washington Post: *"S. Stanley Young, former director of bioinformatics at the National Institute of Statistical Sciences has estimated that for observational studies in the medical field, over 90 percent of the claims fail to replicate"-- that is they cannot be replicated later by more exacting experiments."*[15]

There are also many instances where researchers have read too much into observational studies, and wrongly ignored the stronger evidence from the randomized controlled trials. This was recently demonstrated in a paper published in the American Journal of Clinical Nutrition titled "Belief Beyond the Evidence." The study was meant to focus on bias in research reporting. It used as an example the presumed effect of skipping breakfast on obesity.[16]

Although the scientific literature does not necessarily support a causative role between skipping breakfast and obesity, numerous information sources including blogs, popular health icons, and government agencies have made statements that eating breakfast will help control weight.

When they examined the literature, the study authors found over 90 observational studies that reported associations between breakfast and obesity. But few randomized controlled trials had been conducted looking at breakfast and obesity, and those that had been done had equivocal results. Associations existed, but "mechanistic" studies did not necessarily support a causal relationship. For instance, one common assumption was that skipping breakfast will cause over consumption of energy later in the day, but mechanistic studies often showed no difference in, or even a lower, energy intake after skipping breakfast[17].

This study *"demonstrated that the primary literature often overstates the known relationship between breakfast and obesity. In particular, we showed that there is a substantial use of causative language when describing observational evidence about breakfast and obesity, both when researchers cited others' work as well as when summarizing their own work. In addition, there is evidence that researchers misleadingly cite others' studies to support the presumed effect of breakfast on obesity. Specifically, when authors would cite a study that had results both supporting and refuting the breakfast-obesity hypothesis, authors often would exclude the information against breakfast. Even in their own abstracts, there was a tendency for authors to only make conclusions about breakfast and obesity when the results were in favor of eating breakfast."*[18]

Clearly, the reliability of nutritional studies depends upon the design and quality of the study, regardless of the type of study. Even meta-analyses, at the apex of the pyramid of nutritional studies (see text box below), are frequently criticized as flawed and unreliable.

For instance, a study published in the Journal of the American Medical Association in 2013, titled "Association of All-Cause Mortality With Overweight and Obesity Using Standard Body Mass Index Categories, A Systematic Review and Meta-analysis," contained the counterintuitive findings that people who are overweight live longer[19]. Dr. Walter Willett, at the Harvard School of Public Health, was one of many leading experts to take issue with the conclusions. He was quoted as saying *"This study is really a pile of rubbish and no one should waste their time reading it."* In his book The End of Dieting, Dr. Joel Fuhrman called the study *"essentially worthless."*[20]

The scope of the meta-analysis supposedly included over 3 million people. However, the study was flawed because it looked at the risk of premature death in relation to various body mass index (BMI) categories, without regard for people's health or fitness. It didn't exclude people with chronic disease and former smokers. *"We have a huge amount of other literature showing that people who gain weight or are overweight have increased risk of diabetes, heart disease, stroke, many cancers and many other conditions,"* Willett said[21].

Dr. Fuhrman wrote, *"This is bad science, and because of fatal flaws in the design of the project, it should never have been reported nor published in a major peer-reviewed journal. Especially because other more carefully designed studies, looking at the same issues show the opposite."*[22]

Many authors feel justified in publishing reports of any associations that are found to be statistically significant because they believe the findings are legitimate and warrant attention. There is no doubt that weird results command media attention.

Hierarchy of Nutritional Studies

There are numerous types of nutritional research studies reported in the literature and within each type there is a hierarchy of evidence, with some studies better suited than others to provide more reliable information. The ability of a study to do this rests on the design and quality of the study.

Several design for hierarchy of evidence pyramids exist. A simplified version is shown below:

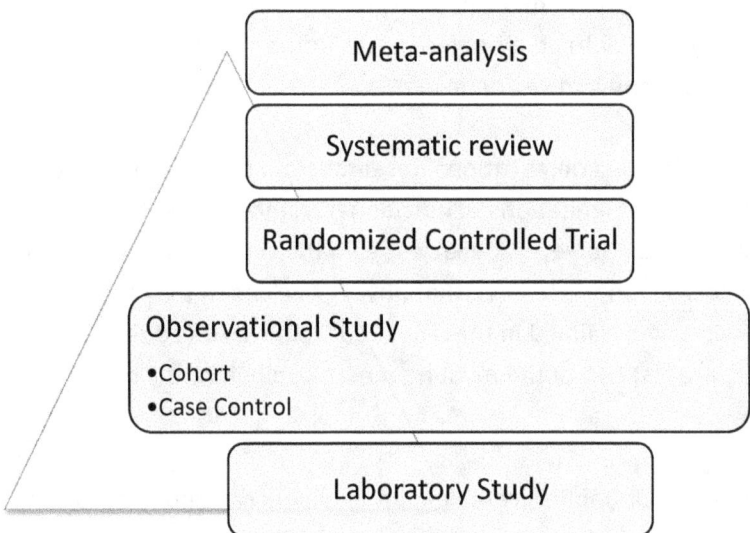

Laboratory studies are performed on cells, tissues, or animals. Studies using isolated cells or tissues usually precede animal-based research. For example, biochemical and molecular nutrition is based on laboratory studies of biochemical metabolism in cell, tissue, and whole animals.

There are different types of observational studies that draw conclusions by comparing subjects against a control group, but the investigator has no control over the experiment. Case-control studies look retrospectively at the characteristics of one group of people who already have a certain health outcome (the cases) and compare them to a similar group of people who do not have the outcome (the controls). Cohort studies prospectively follow large groups of people over a long period of time. Researchers regularly gather information from the people in the study on a wide variety of variables. Once a specified amount of time has elapsed, the characteristics of people in the group are compared to test specific hypotheses.

Randomized Control Trials, (RCT) also follow a group of people over time, but the researchers intervene to watch how a specific change affects the outcome. If participants are randomized via mathematical techniques then the trial is designated as a randomized controlled trial.

A systematic review attempts to consider all published and unpublished material on a specific question. Studies that are judged methodologically sound are then combined quantitatively or qualitatively depending on their similarity.

Meta-analyses combine the data of individual randomized controlled trials and statistically pool it. This

> effectively increases the number of participants that the data was obtained from, thereby increasing the effective sample size. The major drawback to this pooling is that it is dependent on the quality of RCTs that were used[23].

Nutritional studies frequently tend to attract widespread media coverage. Prominent media coverage can be a mixed blessing. The sensationalized reporting of observational study findings that turn out to be merely coincidental or flawed clinical trials that create confusion and public skepticism have caused many to doubt the validity of nutritional research. Single studies have often been widely communicated in the nonscientific media. As information involving sensitive topics surrounding human health surfaces, media normally and commonly formulate opinionated pieces, often with incomplete explanations of study limitations, uncertainty, or conflicting evidence.

It may be that more publicity is focused on nutritional research than other scientific research, but other fields – that do not have the inherent limitations of nutritional sciences – are not totally immune to high-profile, invalid scientific claims. However, debacles seem to occur much more frequently in nutritional science. The surprising reports in 2012 that physicists claimed they found neutrinos traveling faster than light[24], and chemists who claimed in the late 1980s to have solved the world's energy problems with cold fusion[25], are just two of the most memorable, albeit rarely occurring, highly publicized debacles.

And the publication of low-quality or uninterpretable journal papers can and does occur frequently in all types of scientific research[26].

Perhaps nutrition science has greater unmanageable conflicts of interest than other applied sciences. A recent article echoes many past claims that "Big Food" influences the questions that nutrition science asks and the answers that are provided — _or not_[27]. Food companies co-opt experts, and industry-funded studies are renowned for their self-serving attempts to alter federal dietary recommendations[28].

The HHS/USDA Dietary Guidelines for Americans and their forerunner, Dietary Goals for the United States, have been called a battlefield for special interests. The Guidelines' recommendations influence what appears on every "*Nutrition Facts*" label, and are used to determine what types and quantities of food the government purchases and serves in schools, prisons, federal workplaces, and military facilities.

And when they can't influence the questions that nutrition science asks and the answers that are provided, food companies fund messages that raise doubt about studies' findings contrary their interests.

Don't count on the medical community to restore confidence in the credibility of nutritional sciences. According to Dr. Sushrut Jangi, a physician at Beth Israel Deaconess Medical Center, many doctors consider nutritional therapies to be fringe medicine. Even with positive nutritional data, pharmaceuticals continue to trump results from powerful dietary studies[29].

A recent study reported:

"Many U S medical schools still fail to prepare future physicians for everyday nutrition challenges in clinical practice. It cannot be a realistic expectation for physicians to effectively address obesity, diabetes, metabolic syndrome, hospital malnutrition, and many other conditions as long as they are not taught during medical school and residency training how to recognize and treat the nutritional root causes." [30]

However, some doctors are working to address those issues. Recognizing that *"too often, physicians ignore the potential benefits of good nutrition and quickly prescribe medications instead of giving patients a chance to correct their disease through healthy eating and active living,"* some medical doctors have tried to help other physicians understand the potential benefits of a plant-based diet. Working together to create a societal shift toward plant-based nutrition, a group of California doctors wrote, *"Physicians should consider recommending a plant-based diet to all their patients, especially those with high blood pressure, diabetes, cardiovascular disease, or obesity."* [31]

As recently as 2008 a study reported that while some physicians do hold positive views about the importance of nutrition, most primary care providers are not adequately trained to provide nutritional counseling[32].

Resolve to Overcome Barriers to Healthful Eating

The Standard American Diet, which is responsible for epidemic levels of obesity, hypertension, heart disease and diabetes, may owe its deep entrenchment in the fabric of our society to the confusion created by nutritional science. But that doesn't provide sufficient reason to disparage the validity of an entire body of knowledge, throw caution to the wind and eat all of the junk food within reach. Remember the adage, "More people commit suicide with the fork than any other weapon." We have to exercise self control, act responsibly, become informed, and acquire at least an elementary understanding of nutritional principles.

Sound health advice regarding nutrition and supplements is generally based on research that evolves over time. Revolutionary findings are <u>rare</u> and limited to arranging or re-arranging some pieces of an extraordinarily complex puzzle – the molecular basis of human nutrition and diet-disease relations. The peer-reviewed literature is the one and only place where new facts are published. Everything else is just someone's re-interpretation or opinion about those facts. Note, however, that peer review <u>per se</u> is not a guarantor of reliable knowledge, and the state of research might be too ambiguous to provide meaningful knowledge.

Laypeople have to learn how to ignore the food misinformation appearing in various popular media— TV, newspapers, general consumer magazines, and the tabloid press — such as weight loss regimens, megavitamins, and food supplements, to name a few. Don't fall prey to the ready availability and convenience of supplements and the ubiquitous usage of food additives. Don't ignore scientific data but treat all studies, models, and predictions with a degree of skepticism. And resolve to stay informed and transform the conflicting information into useful knowledge.

That advice may strike you as time consuming. It can be very time consuming and possibly frustrating. There is an easier approach: A time honored way to make informed decisions is to seek advice from experts. In this case we suggest that you obtain and compare the opinions of multiple sources including your physician and authoritative online resources such as the Nutrition Source at the Harvard School of Public Health[33], the Linus Pauling Institute[34], the Mayo Clinic[35], and Berkeley Wellness[36].

Try to find the best evidence that is available, learn the relevant facts, carefully weigh the benefits, risks, and drawbacks (including, e.g. the inconvenience of foregoing the convenience and comfort of poor food choices), and decide which plant based dietary option (or options) to choose. Select from among the alternatives that appear to be best for you. Then eat what tastes best to you.

No Magic Bullets Now and for the Foreseeable Future

There are people inclined to ignore warnings about unhealthful foods, hoping to take pills to fend off the harmful consequences of poor choices[37].

For example, many people who take Statins continue to eat excessive amounts of high fat foods, adding more cholesterol to their bodies, and expecting the pills to act as magic bullets. Taking Statins is no excuse to continue eating a diet high in fat.[38]

Similarly, wishful expectations can fuel harmful rationalizations. Examples include the obese and borderline obese people who continue to eat too much and exercise too little because of news reports concerning obesity vaccines or a vaccine that could prevent the development of Type-2 diabetes[39].

The prospect of a new vaccine is not a valid justification to continue to make poor choices in your diet and lifestyle.

Chapter Nine includes a number of incisive questions to ask about food and health claims and announcements to help you determine their credibility and how important the results are for you personally. Energetic readers with some science training who are inclined to scrutinize the technical literature may want consult the references in Chapter Ten, where there are several web addresses for articles that provide guidance for critically reviewing nutrition studies and understanding the standards for evidence-based recommendations.

In this book we will briefly discuss the nutritarian, vegan, vegetarian, and flexitarian diets styles, which are four of the leading options that are consistent with the best dietary information available today. By the time you have finished reading Chapter Five you will be ready to choose any one of the four options, or you may elect to step through any or all of them in a serial fashion.

A four step ladder, for example, might begin with a flexitarian diet[40], a plant-based diet that occasionally (up to 10% of calories –Fuhrman's version) includes meat, fish, poultry, eggs, and dairy in small quantities. The next step could be a vegetarian diet, a plant-based diet that excludes meat, fish, and poultry. Alternatively, there are vegetarian diets that exclude meat, fish, and poultry but allow consumption of dairy products and eggs, or permit dairy but not eggs, or eggs but not dairy products.

From vegetarian diets you could progress to a vegan diet, a plant-based diet that excludes all animal products (excluding also foods of animal product origin, e.g. honey[41] and gelatin), but does allow for the consumption of processed foods.

The last step on the ladder might be the nutritarian diet[42], a plant-based diet that emphasizes greens, beans, onions, mushrooms, berries, and seeds, with a focus on the micronutrient content of foods, but allows limited amounts (prescribed safe levels) of animal products. According to the diet's author, *"The more nutrient-dense food you consume, the more you'll be satisfied with fewer calories, and the less you'll crave fat and high-calorie foods."*

Finally, with the knowledge and experience that you have acquired, you are still free to fashion your own healthful diet, personalized to your needs and tastes. The path you take will depend upon your goal (destination) and which diet you can learn to enjoy and follow faithfully.

If you haven't yet determined the goal or goals for your transition to a healthful, plant based diet now is a good time to do so. Do you want to lose weight, address current health issues, reduce the risk of certain diseases, improve the quality of your life, or try to live longer? The answer should help you choose the best path forward.

This is a voyage that matters. Make a resolution to take the journey and a commitment to see it through.

Food for Thought

1. How does the controversial nature of nutritional science affect: the education of our nation's school children and schoolteachers; the education and licensing of dieticians; the home economics (aka family and consumer sciences) curricula in schools and colleges, or the food sciences curricula at universities?

2. The congressionally mandated, federal Dietary Guidelines are supposed to serve as the vehicle whereby two federal agencies, USDA and HHS, speak with one voice on nutrition issues for the health of Americans. Yet critics argue that the Guidelines reflect the influence of special interests. Are private economic interests less likely to influence the combined voices of the USDA or HHS?

3. It is widely reported that healthful foods can also reverse certain diseases or disabilities, protect against dementia, increase life expectancy[43], help you lose excess weight, and reduce your medical expenses. However, laboratory studies with insects and worms showed that while dietary restrictions

contributed to longer lives, the animals that lived longer had the same portion of their lives being healthy but added more time being frail. Researchers argue that if applied to humans, life-extension ideas such as caloric restriction would likely lead to unsustainable healthcare costs[44]. Should future research funds be focused on healthspan improvements or lifespan extension?

4. The current global population of over 7 billion is said to be several times higher than a sustainable level, depending on the standard of living that is used for reference. Unrestrained growth and advances in medicine and agriculture are major contributing factors. Does progress in dietary disease prevention contribute to or conflict with sustainable population growth?

5. The FDA in 1996 approved a food additive that offers the prospect of food with zero calories, zero grams of cholesterol and zero grams of fat. But the side effects included cramps, gas and loose bowels and hampered ability of the body to absorb essential vitamins. Why haven't food technologists created a dietary fat replacement with no undesirable side effects?

6. For which of these foods do you expect growing food demands: functional foods like oatmeal; snack and convenience food with high protein and fiber; foods with soy protein, algae protein, or insect protein; coconut or palm oil; nuts or seeds; amaranth, quinoa, or millet; whole grains or sprouted grains; low- and no-calorie sweeteners; real fruits and vegetables; ready-to-eat steamed and peeled vegetables; food products with marijuana?

7. Resolve the conflicts in following statements about infant formula and breastfeeding:

> A. A heralded innovation in pediatric nutrition was the development of the caloric method of infant feeding which led to the large-scale adoption of a single infant formula. This required cooperation with industry and ultimately led to the development of life-saving specialty formulas for various disease states including inborn errors of metabolism[45].

> B. Currently, infant formula has a profound effect on the number of mothers who breastfeed their infants. Breastfeeding rates in the United States have decreased significantly in the 21st century, resulting in serious health issues that include atopy (the genetic tendency to develop allergic diseases), diabetes mellitus, and childhood obesity. Research suggests that breastfeeding prevents adverse health conditions, whereas formula-feeding is linked with their development[46].

Chapter Two: Weights and Measures

"It requires good judgment, and this can be applied only when there is sound comprehension not only of the science involved, but also of the ways in which it is being applied, and, more subtly, of the ways in which it is likely to be applied in the future." – Vannevar Bush[47]

For over 150 years, researchers have conducted body composition studies and assessments and tried to develop techniques to predict health and disease states. There are several measures commonly used to measure or classify healthy bodies and healthy foods. They include food calories, body mass index, percent body fat, and nutrient density. There are also procedures and devices that are employed to estimate body fat. Underwater weighing, whole-body air displacement, skinfold caliper measurements, and dual-energy x-ray absorptiometry are common examples. In this chapter we will discuss their usage, validity and potential value for individual users.

Calories Count

The energy in food is stored as chemical energy, which is contained in the chemical bonds of food molecules. A food Calorie is a unit of energy.

Note about food Calories

In physics and chemistry calories are written with a lower case letter "c" but food calories, which are equal to 1000 physical calories, are written with the upper case letter "C." So one food Calorie is actually 1000 physical calories. The common convention in the literature of food and nutrition is to write food calories with the lower case letter "c" even though each is 1000 calories. However, government agencies and other institutions frequently use "kcal."

Some of the energy in food is released during chemical reactions that occur with digestion when chemical bonds break and oxidation occurs. Different foods store different amounts of chemical energy, and different people will process the same amount of caloric intake in different ways. The same person can process the same amount of caloric intake at different times in different ways. For example, given the same caloric intake, different people will store different amounts of calories as fat, and a person can store different amounts of calories as fat at different times of intake. Digestion and appetite are very complicated linked processes. You may want to pause to read simplified descriptions in the text boxes that follow. For reasons of clarity and brevity we have limited the details to include components that are directly relevant to the discussions in this book. For example, mention is made of only a half dozen the two dozen gut hormones that are identified in the literature.

The Molecular Basis of Digestion is Very Complicated and Not Yet Totally Understood

The chemical process begins in the mouth but varies somewhat for different kinds of food. The three sets of salivary glands produce saliva, which moistens food and begins the digestion of carbohydrates. Salivary amylase, an enzyme in saliva, splits complex carbohydrates into simple carbohydrates.

The stomach contains hydrochloric acid and digestive enzymes that continue the chemical digestion of food that began in the mouth. Protein digestion begins in the stomach with pepsin an active protein-digesting enzyme.

Absorption begins in the stomach with simple molecules like water and alcohol being absorbed directly into the bloodstream. The mixture of food, liquid, and digestive juice is referred to as chyme.

Chyme passes out of the stomach into the first section of the small intestine, the duodenum, where it is mixed with bile salts from the liver that help digest fats and fat soluble vitamins (vitamins A,D,E,K), plus enzymes from the pancreas that help digest carbohydrates and fats, and bicarbonate from the pancreas that neutralizes stomach acid. Next, the chyme passes through the jejunum, the second part of the small intestine, where about 90% of the proteins, carbohydrates, vitamins, and minerals are absorbed.

Lastly, the chyme passes through the ileum, the third section of the small intestine, where water, bile salts, and vitamin B_{12}, are absorbed before entering the large intestine. In the large intestine, fluids and electrolytes, including sodium and potassium are absorbed and dietary fibers are fermented to produce short chain fatty acids, which are also absorbed.

Both insulin and glucagon are secreted from the pancreas, and thus are referred to as pancreatic endocrine hormones. Problems in the production or regulation of pancreatic hormones will cause complications related to blood sugar imbalance. Diabetes, the most common disorder of the endocrine system, occurs when blood sugar levels in the body consistently stay above normal. It is a disease brought on by either the body's inability to make insulin (type 1 diabetes) or by the body not responding to the effects of insulin (type 2 diabetes).

The digestible carbohydrates are broken down into sugar, which enters the blood stream. With rising blood sugar levels the pancreas produces insulin, which prompts cells to absorb the blood sugar for energy and storage. When the blood sugar levels fall the pancreas makes glucagon, a hormone that signals the liver to release stored sugar. The maintenance of blood sugar levels is especially important to provide the brain with the steady supply of glucose it needs to function.

Food and the Brain

Gut–brain interactions control appetite and satiety through neuronal and hormonal signals. The brain receives signals from the gastrointestinal tract through sensory nerves and the circulation.

The brain processes food-related signals about gastrointestinal contents from the vagus nerves located in the stomach and intestines. Those different signals intersect in the hindbrain where together they act to <u>reduce</u> further food intake. For example, the gut peptide cholecystokinin (CCK) is a hormone that activates vagal signals that contribute to satiation. Cholecystokinin was the first gut-secreted peptide to be identified as a satiety factor. Subsequently, many other peptides, receptors and intracellular pathways have been revealed, mostly promoting reduction of food intake.

Research suggests that leptin, another hormone, amplifies the CCK signals to enhance the feeling of fullness. Leptin and insulin are released in the hypothalamus and reward centers of the brain to suppress appetite and inhibit eating pleasure. Other research suggests that leptin also interacts with the neurotransmitter dopamine in the brain to produce a feeling of pleasure after eating.

Additionally, the brain processes other sensory signals from the gut. The only known appetite stimulating is ghrelin. Researchers have postulated three different pathways for the appetite-inducing effects of the hormone ghrelin. First, after release into the bloodstream by the stomach, ghrelin may cross the blood brain barrier and bind to its receptors in the hypothalamus. Second, ghrelin may reach the brain through the vagal nerve and the visceral sensory nucleus of the hindbrain. Third, ghrelin is produced locally in the hypothalamus, where it may directly affect the various hypothalamic nuclei[48].

Eating slowly allows this intricate hormonal cross-talk system enough time to work.

More recently intestinal microbiota have been linked to obesity and metabolic disorders, but there are still many controversial issues on the physiological and pathological implications of the gut microbiota and host relationships that need to be addressed to establish the precise role of intestinal microbiota in human health[49].

Food provides powerful visual, smell and taste signals which can override satiety and stimulate eating. The abundance of low-cost, palatable, energy-dense processed foods and their ability to activate central nervous system centers that drive food preference and overeating is frequently cited as an important factor in the obesity epidemic.

Learning what happens when sensory signals override the satiety signals and overstimulate the rewards system in the brain is a topic of active research. It has been hypothesized that an inbalance might contribute to obesity[50].

The digestion of food requires about ten percent of a human's total energy expenditure. Most of the daily energy expenditure occurs as a result of basal metabolism – the minimal amount of energy necessary to maintain respiration, circulation, and other vital body functions while fasting and at total

---

Energy Balance

Humans acquire energy through the intake of food and beverages, and expend energy through physical activity, their resting metabolic rate (RMR), and the thermic effect of food (TEF).

The RMR is responsible for 60–75 percent of the total calories burned each day. The RMR is the energy expenditure required for maintaining normal body functions and to physiologically regulate its inner environment. The RMR is proportional to body mass, in particular fat-free mass. The energy required to digest, absorb, transport, and store the food consumed is called the thermic effect of food (TEF). It typically accounts for 8–10 % of daily energy expenditure.

The energy expended due to physical activity includes voluntary exercise, shivering, postural control, and voluntary movement. It is the most variable component of energy expenditure. The more sedentary the individual is, the lower the effect of physical activity. The decline in energy expenditure that occurs with advancing age is mainly the results of declining lean body mass, which reduces TEF and physical activity.

Disturbances in energy balance cause changes in body mass. The timeframe over which this occurs varies between individuals and may explain the large inter-individual response to weight-loss interventions. A positive energy balance, in which energy intake exceeds expenditure causes weight gain, with 60–80 % of the resulting weight gain being attributable to body fat. In negative energy balance, when energy expenditure exceeds intake, the resulting loss in body mass is also accounted for by 60–80 % body fat.

It is commonly assumed that energy intake and energy expenditure can be independently modified, through changes in food intake and physical activity, to achieve energy balance. However, energy input and expenditure are interdependent and regulated at several levels. This involves a complex physiologic control system, which includes afferent neural and hormonal signals reaching the hypothalamus, with resultant efferent projections of the autonomic nervous system innervating the muscle, viscera, and adipose tissue. (Afferent means towards; efferent means away from)

As a result of this physiologic control, components of energy intake and expenditure cannot be altered without compensatory changes in the other. The components of energy balance influence each other and serve to maintain a constant body mass. For example, when calorie intake is reduced, the body responds by both stimulating hunger and reducing the RMR so that less energy is expended. Similarly, an increase in physical activity could result in increased hunger or reductions in physical activity at other times during the day.

The compensation in response to positive energy balance seems to be weaker that the compensation in response to negative energy balance[51].

rest. The remaining twenty percent is due to physical activities. The direct effects of physical activity on energy expenditure are relatively small when placed in the context of total daily energy demands[52]. You will gain weight when you consume more calories than your burn and when you burn fewer calories than you eat. A popular (but highly oversimplified) example, is that a person could gain about a pound of body weight in a week by consuming 3500 excess calories, or lose a pound by burning 3500 excess calories. Exercise will burn calories, but clearly it is much easier and more expeditious to eat an extra 500 calories each day than to burn an additional 500 calories per day through exercise (a competitive eater can consume 2,000 calories/minute but an elite athletes can only burn 20 calories/minute). The more weight you lose the more difficult it will be to lose additional weight. And not all of the weight lost will necessarily come from body fat. Although health-related outcomes are often improved with the loss of body weight due to declines in body fat, skeletal muscle mass is also lost and may account for 25% or more of the total body weight loss[53].

It is important to monitor your weight during the period when you are changing your eating habits so that you can control your consumption of calories. You should consistently check your weight with the same accurate scale at the same time(s) of day wearing the same amount of clothing, preferably none.

Table 1 and the graph for Table 1 show compressed versions for an example of a spreadsheet used to graph body weight recorded daily each month. In this case provisions are included for recording weight before and after each of three daily meals. Measuring body weight that frequently is not practical, doing so is unnecessary and the measurements are subject to several different kinds of errors. However, daily monitoring can be a useful tool.

	1-Jan	2-Jan	....	31-Jan
Before Breakfast				
After Breakfast				
Before Lunch				
After Lunch				
Before Dinner				
After Dinner				
Average				

Table 1

The best single reading to monitor is the weight before breakfast because it isn't subject to abrupt changes due to eating, exercise, or other activities. You can learn to control your weight by monitoring the pattern of weight changes and adjusting ("titrating") your eating, drinking, resting, and exercise routines. Monitoring daily weight changes might also help motivate you stay the course.

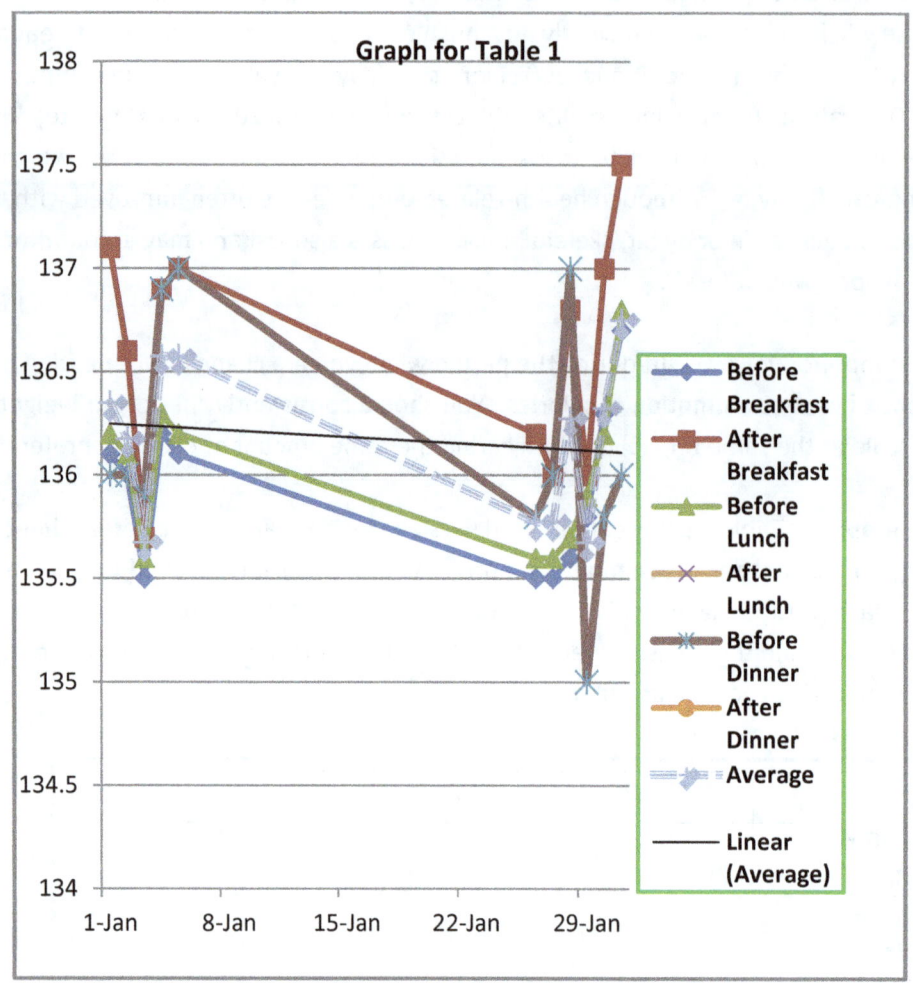

Similarly, it is important to be aware of the calories that you consume during the period when you are changing your eating habits. The exact amount of calories contained in the food is not practical to measure and not even important. It is the <u>relative</u> caloric values of alternative foods that are important and of interest. For example, labels or tables might list the calories in a cube of refined white sugar as 9 calories in 0.1 oz, and 4 calories in a carrot weighing 0.4 oz. So sugar has about 90 calories per ounce and carrots have about 10 calories per ounce, for a ration of 9 to 1. If you know the approximate number of calories that you consume per day and you know approximately how many calories are contained in the food you eat, you will be better able to control your weight loss or gain during the period your eating habits are changing by adjusting the number of servings of sugar or carrots.

Using sugar cubes in another elementary example: If you normally do not eat sugar cubes but somehow get into the habit of eating the equivalent of 100 sugar cubes a day, your will surely gain weight, and if you don't want to continue to gain weight you should quit eating the sugar cubes. For obvious reasons, it would not be a good idea to continue to eat 100 sugar cubes a day and reduce your daily consumption of other food by approximately 900 calories. (If eating 100 sugar cubes a day seems like a ridiculous example, perhaps eating two, 16 oz. Starbucks white chocolate mocha drinks or a couple Potbelly oatmeal chocolate chip cookies are better 900 calorie equivalent snacks to visualize.)

An interesting, user-friendly, and entertaining computer model was recently published online by the NIH[54]. The model attempts to simulate how factors such as diet and exercise can alter metabolism over time and thereby lead to changes of weight and body fat. An image of the input is shown below.

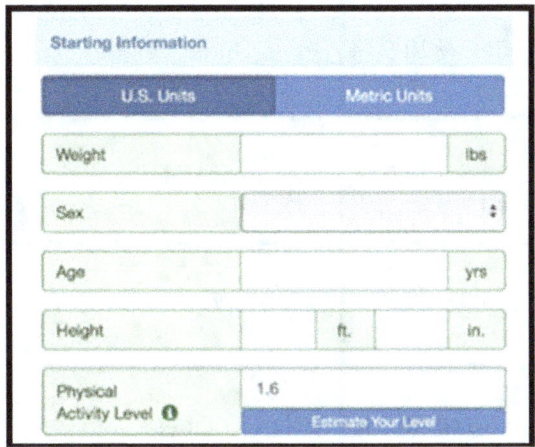

Input for NIH Body Weight Planner[55]

For some people, especially obese individuals, the issue of weight loss and weight regain is much more complex than trying to manage a simple energy balance. Lifestyle intervention can successfully induce weight loss even in obese persons, at least temporarily. However, there currently is no way to quantitatively estimate the changes of diet or physical activity required to prevent weight regain for obese people.

Body Mass Index (BMI)

Body Mass Index (BMI) is a popular measure that is over 180 years old. The concept was invented in 1835 and was referred to as the Quetelet Index[56]. The index didn't become popular until it was resurrected from obscurity in 1972 by Ancel Keys who published a paper in the Journal of Chronic Diseases in which he used the term body mass index[57].

BMI is presented here because it is frequently mentioned or discussed in publications concerning weight loss, and nutrition.

The BMI is like density, which is mass per unit volume, except BMI compares weight with height squared. Knowing your height and weight you can determine your body mass index.
BMI is calculated as:

BMI = (weight in kilograms)/(height in meters squared), or

BMI = (weight in pounds x 703)/(height in inches squared)

BMI is frequently used as a screening tool to indicate whether a person's weight is high, normal, or too low. It is commonly associated with body fatness.

One established interpretation of BMI values associated with weight categories for adults 20 years old and older, regardless of gender, body types, and ages is shown in the following table[58].

BMI	WEIGHT STATUS
Below 18.5	Underweight
18.5 – 24.9	Normal or Healthy Weight
25.0 – 29.9	Overweight
30.0 and Above	Obese

If your BMI is less than 18.5, it falls within the underweight range.
If your BMI is 18.6 to 24.9, it falls within the normal or *"Healthy Weight"* range.
If your BMI is 25.0 to 29.9, it falls within the overweight range.
If your BMI is 30.0 or higher, it falls within the obese range.

Both the BMI formula and the BMI numerical values for the four categories have been criticized as antiquated and flawed.

Professor Nick Trefethen, an Oxford University mathematician, showed that the formula's exponent should be 2.5 instead of 2 in order to better approximate the actual sizes and shapes of human bodies. He pointed out that the traditional formula makes tall people seem fatter and short people seem to have less body fat. Another mathematician suggested that the exponent should be between 2.3 and 2.7. Additionally, the results of using the MI ranges in the original formula can classify people who are actually overweight as normal or healthy. Dr. Joel Fuhrman states that the maximum acceptable Healthy Weight is 22.5, not 25, and that the flaw in the classification condones feeling OK about carrying a lot of excess fat[59].

Professor Trefethen has proposed a more accurate BMI formula[60]:

$$BMI = 1.3 \times weight(kg) / height(m)^{2.5} = 5734 \times weight(lb)/height(in)^{2.5}$$

[The BMI formula is not applicable to children and teenagers who are still growing, lactating or pregnant women, bodybuilders and athletes with large muscle mass, elderly, frail, and certain sick people, and it does not account for racial differences. There are BMI calculators for children and teens, 2 – 19 years old.]

Even this newer, more accurate BMI formula is just a ballpark calculation that should not be used to establish healthy weights for individuals. BMI overestimates body fat in persons who are very muscular and can underestimate body fat in persons who have lost muscle mass (e.g., the elderly).

Central Adiposity (Obesity)

Central adiposity is the accumulation of fat in the lower torso around the abdominal area. Central adiposity includes both subcutaneous fat that sits under the skin, and intra-abdominal visceral fat that surrounds the internal organs in the peritoneal cavity. Some researchers believe that visceral adipose tissue may represent a pathological adipose tissue depot, which accumulates when subcutaneous depots are overwhelmed or otherwise unavailable for storage[61].

Intra-abdominal fat has two compartments: visceral and retroperitoneal, but in the literature, retroperitoneal and peritoneal fat depots are quantified together as visceral fat, to study their relationships to cardio-metabolic diseases[62]. Researchers argue that retroperitoneal fat area should be included in the measurement of visceral fat for cardio-metabolic studies in humans[63].

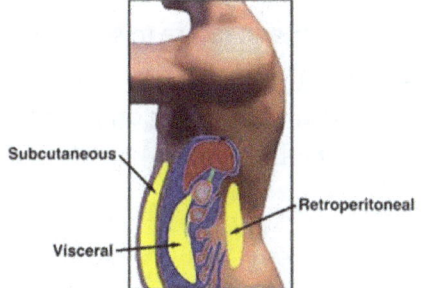

Central adiposity increases the risk for cardiovascular and other diseases independent of obesity. Clinicians use the waist circumference as a measure of central adiposity. Men with waist circumferences greater than 102 cm (>40 inches) and women with waist circumferences greater than 88 cm (>35 inches) are at increased risk for cardiovascular disease. The waist circumference thresholds are not reliable for patients with a BMI greater than 35 kg/m^2; waist circumference has little added predictive power of disease risk beyond that of BMI[64].

Waist circumference is a better estimate of intra-abdominal fat, the dangerous internal fat which coats the organs. According to NIH, *"Waist circumference is the most practical anthropometric measurement for assessing a patient's abdominal fat content before and during weight loss treatment*[65]. In children and adolescents, waist circumference is the best simple index of fat distribution, since it is least affected by gender, race, and overall adiposity[66].

A recent study found that persons with normal-weight central obesity had the worst long-term survival. For example, a man with a normal BMI (22 kg/m^2) and central obesity had greater total mortality risk than one with similar BMI but no central obesity, and this man had twice the mortality risk of participants who were overweight or obese according to BMI only. Women with normal-weight central obesity also had a higher mortality risk than those with similar BMI but no central obesity. Expected survival estimates were consistently lower for those with central obesity when age and BMI were controlled for[67].

You cannot establish an accurate healthy weight from height and weight BMI measurements alone. However, that hasn't stopped people from continuing to rely on it, including the medical doctors who routinely use it for diagnosis, as an indicator of health status and disease risk, and to establish goals for patients. At an individual level, BMI can be used as a screening tool but it is not diagnostic of the body fatness or health of an individual[68]. BMI is only sensitive to weight changes and cannot discriminate among sources of weight changes, such as hydration.

The adoption of a healthy diet and increasing physical activity can result in significant improvement in cardiorespiratory fitness, which could occur independent of weight changes. In such instances even reduction in waist circumference (and abdominal fat) will not be reflected in the change of BMI. Moreover, when you lose weight through exercise and proper nutrition the first fat to go is the fat at the waist line. People with normal weight (i.e., normal BMI) and excess pounds around the middle may not have as much muscle mass as people without belly fat, these individuals may benefit from an exercise routine that includes strength and resistance training in addition to aerobic activity[69].

Inadvisably, BMI may be used by the reader as a measure to set a target goal, if weight loss is one of your goals. But if you are an adult weight is the only variable parameter in the BMI formula, since your height is not going to change. Why go through the trouble of performing calculations that include exponents or spend time plugging your weight and height into an online calculator when you can just track your weight with a scale?

Percent Body Fat

Since the BMI formula cannot even distinguish between lean body mass and body fat, it is clearly not a measure of body fat. Conceptually, percent body fat should be better suited than BMI for establishing a healthy weight for an individual.

The lean body mass is comprised of structural and functional elements in cells, water, muscle, bone, heart, liver, kidneys, and other organs. Body fat includes essential fat and storage fat. Essential fat is necessary for normal physiological functioning (e.g. nerve conduction). Storage fat constitutes the body's fat reserves. The storage fat that is of most concern is the visceral fat component of abdominal fat that surrounds your internal organs because it is the most strongly correlated with metabolic disease risk factors, and the subcutaneous component of abdominal fat because it is the most highly correlated with insulin resistance. So it is not surprising that some experts believe that body-fat percentage may be a better measure of your risk of weight-related diseases than BMI[70].

If the more appropriate measure is percent body fat then how much body fat is healthy? The American Council on Exercise has published the following ranges[71]:

Body Fat Percentage Categories

Classification	Women (% Fat)	Men (% Fat)
Essential Fat	10-12%	2-4%
Athletes	14-20%	6-13%
Fitness	21-24%	14-17%
Acceptable	25-31%	18-25%
Obese	32% +	25% +

Once again, *"essential fat"* is supposed to be the minimum amount of fat necessary for basic physical and physiological health. This is a frequently cited body fat chart.

Other organizations have published body fat charts that include other categories, such as *"ideal,"* other factors such as *"age,"* and even different estimates for people who participate in different sports. There is a lot of controversy over what amount of body fat is optimal for overall health.

Medical researchers have attempted to establish definitive body fat ranges but have not yet succeeded in doing so because they lack the information needed to directly associate percentage body fat with morbidity and mortality.

Although body fat percentages are more appropriate measures of potential health risks than BMI, and body fat measurements can be more accurate, the medical profession continues to use the well established BMI because they claim it is said to be more practical for clinical settings. <u>Accurate</u> body fat measurement can be expensive and is generally not readily as available as BMI.

<u>Body Fat Measurement</u>

Body fat is the most variable constituent of the body. There are a number of methods commonly used to estimate an individual's body fat. All are just very rough estimates of an individual's body fat. There is no true reference standard for the measurement of body fat. Even the popular reference model, the so-called <u>four compartment model</u> ((1) fat mass, 2) total body water, 3) bone mineral matter, and 4) residual/protein)), against which some of these methods are compared is just an estimate of the actual amounts.

Additionally, all body fat measures are subject to some degree of inaccuracy both for one-time measurements and multiple measurements for tracking body fat changes over time. All are based on some assumptions, which have not been completely validated. Some are more accurate or precise than others. A critical review of popular body fat measures was recently published online by *Weightology Weekly*[72].

> **Multi-compartment models**
>
> With multi-compartment models, the multiple compartments of the fat-free mass (water, bone mineral, and residual/protein) are individually estimated, allowing for calculation of the density of fat-free mass, and that increases the precision with which body composition can be estimated. Because of these advantages, the four compartment model is often referred to as the gold standard against which other techniques are "validated."

Body fat measurement techniques have been used to help individuals set baseline values for body composition and establish future goals. Several of the most commonly discussed methods are examined below. Knowledge of their limitations should provide you with realistic expectations concerning their usefulness.

Underwater Weighing (hydrostatic weighing or hydrodensitometry)

As you might have suspected, this method depends upon Archimedes principle. The story goes that Archimedes discovered the principle while he was at a public bath thinking about how to detect a fake gold crown – a crown composed of gold plus another metal. Gold has a greater density than any metal that might have been used to create an alloy to dilute it. So the problem became a matter of finding the density of an irregular shaped object whose volume could not easily be measured. To solve that problem today we might weigh the crown in air and again when it is immersed in water. Next, use Archimedes equation that states his principle that the buoyant force equals the weight of the fluid displaced and that allows us to calculate the volume of the crown:

weight in air – weight in water = volume x (specific gravity of water)

[Recall also that the specific gravity of water is equal to 1 and the specific gravity of any substance is equal to the weight density]

So the volume is the only unknown in the equation and after calculating the volume we use the equation

Density$_{(crown)}$ = weight in air / volume

to calculate the density of the crown, which would have been less than the density of a crown made of pure gold if it were composed of a gold alloy. In the story of Archimedes the gold crown was found to be a gold-silver alloy.

Similarly, the process for this measurement is to first determine the density of a human body, then plug the density measurement in a formula that is supposed to calculate the percentage of body fat (by analogy it is equivalent to the silver in the crown). The body density is calculated from a formula:

Body density = dry weight / [((dry weight – wet weight) / water density) – RV – 0.1)]

The units for weight are expressed in kg and RV is in liters (L). RV is the residual lung volume. The 0.1 represents the estimated volume (L) of gas trapped in the gastrointestinal tract.

The body density (D) can be converted to percent body fat (%BF) using either the Siri equation or the Brozek equation (the Brozek equation is said to be more accurate than Siri for older adults).[73]

Siri: %BF = [(4.95 / Body Density) – 4.50] x 100

Brozek: %BF = [(4.570 / Body Density) – 4.142] x 100

This step is the source of the largest errors. The body fat equations erroneously assume the density of the fat-free mass is the same for different people, including lean, muscular individuals and obese individuals, and people of different ethnicity. Additionally, fat-free mass includes everything that is not fat, including your organs, muscle, bone, and body water. Hence a change in body water will affect the composition of fat-free mass. Weight loss or weight gain, other than fat, between measurements also contributes to error.

Since this method divides the body into just two components, fat and fat-free mass, it is classified as a two compartment model. The measurement error for this test is generally reported by various sources to be very low when compared to other two compartment methods with the exception of DEXA (a three compartment model discussed below). However, when compared to the four compartment model, the error rate for individuals can be 5%-6% body fat on a given day (for a one-time measurement) and because weight changes can alter the calculation of fat free mass the error, compared to the four compartment model, the error can be twice as high when tracking an individual's body fat changes over time[74].

Air Displacement Plethysmography

Air-displacement plethysmography, such as Bod Pod, is similar to underwater weighing because it measures the air displaced by an individual to determine their body density. Body weight and volume are used to calculate density, and body density is then used to calculate percent body fat.

This technique has more variables that can affect error rates than underwater weighing. A study that compared it to the four compartment model reported an error for one-time measurements of up to 11% in individuals. It also is subject to much greater errors than underwater weighing when tracking changes in body fat for individuals over time. When compared to the four compartment model, the study found essentially no agreement between the two methods[75].

Skinfold Caliper Measurements

This method attempts to estimate body fat percentage starting with the measurement of the thickness of one or more skin folds at specific spots on the body using a body fat caliper. Those measurements are plugged into an equation that includes the subject's age, to calculate the individual's body density. The body density is then used in a body fat percentage equation like, for example, the Siri equation. Alternatively, the skinfold measurements can be compared to a chart, which includes provisions for age and gender, to arrive at an estimate of body fat percentage.

The test is very much dependent on the person doing the testing, the quality of the calipers used, and the equation that is used to predict body density, particularly if the equation wasn't specifically developed for the subject's race, age, and gender. Be aware that skinfold equations are based on data derived from hydrostatic weighing measurements, hence the error rates will be compounded. And, as in the case of hydrostatic weight measurements, errors can occur as the result of changes in body weight when attempting to measure a change in body fat over time.

Compared to the four compartment model, high individual error rates for one-time measurements have been reported, ranging from +10% - 15%. When measuring change in body fat over time, individual error rates under-predicted the body fat percentage by approximately 5% and over-predicted the body fat percentage by approximately 3%. Surprisingly, skinfold measurements did much better than might have been expected when tracking changes in individuals over time.

The skinfold measurement is not an accurate way to predict body fat changes. However, the devices for measuring skinfolds are inexpensive and readily available. The calipers could be useful, in the hands of a skilled operator, for just tracking the changes in skinfold thickness over long time intervals (quarterly, semi-annually, or annually). One assessment concluded, *"The best application of Skinfold Calipers is to determine if subcutaneous fat is increasing or decreasing, but not for predicting total body fat[76]."* Also keep in mind that skinfold measurement does not measure deep belly fat, which is strongly correlated with risk factors[77].

Dual energy X-ray absortiometry (DEXA)

DEXA is said to be based on a three-compartment model that divides the body into total body mineral, fat-free soft (lean) mass, and fat tissue mass. It works by measuring the body's absorbance of x-rays at two different energy levels. By measuring the absorption of each beam into parts of the body, the device can estimate the bone mineral density, lean body mass, and fat mass, which have different absorption properties.

A critical review argues that DXA is not really a three-compartment technology, because it estimates bone in every pixel and in 50% of pixels guesses the proportions of fat and non-bone fat free mass[78].

Although DEXA is not subject to errors caused by variations in bone density among different ethnicities, it is susceptible to hydration error that can be a problem for comparing different ethnicities or body types and DEXA is subject to numerous other sources of errors. Hydration error can also be a problem when measuring changes over time. And the accuracy of this method can be affected by sex, size, fatness, and health issues.

Different DEXA machines can produce different results due to hardware and software variability and errors. Error rates for individuals average about 5%, but can be as high as 10%, and error rates for body fat changes over time average about 5%. Although DEXA is based on a quasi-three compartment model, its error rates are not better than hydrostatic weighing, which is based on a two compartment model, and can even be worse.

While DEXA is the only method discussed here that is capable of body fat distribution analysis and it is the only scanner FDA-approved to quantify dangerous deep belly fat, which is important for health assessments, it requires whole body exposure to low-dose radiation, and is regarded as too impractical and expensive to be recommended for our purposes[79].

Bioelectrical Impedance Analysis

Fat-free mass contains mostly water (72%), while fat contains very little water. Thus, fat-free mass will have less resistance to an electric current than fatty tissue. Bioelectrical impedance analysis (BIA) measures the electrical impedance, or opposition to flow, of electric current, which provides an estimate of total body water (TBW). Using values of TBW derived from BIA along with height and weight, one can then estimate fat-free mass and body fat (adiposity). BIA values are affected by numerous variables including body position, hydration status, consumption of food and beverages, ambient air and skin temperature, recent physical activity, and conductance of the examining table[80].

The equation used to generate estimates is usually based on the results of tests performed on a large number of people using underwater weighing instead of the more accurate four compartment model. Basing estimates on data that are derived from methods that are themselves subject to error (recall that the error rate for underwater weighing rate for individuals can be 5%-6% body fat) compounds the errors that occur in the BIA measures.

BIA readings can be greatly affected by variables like hydration levels. Since it is difficult to control the path of the electric current, the devices can miss entire sections of the body. When compared with the four compartment model, one study found the error rate for individuals can be +/- 8% body fat. The disagreement between BIA and the four compartment model ranged from minus 3.6% to 4.8% in one study to minus 8.1% to 7.9% in another for measuring body fat change over time[81].

A report titled "Bioelectrical impedance analysis in body composition measurement: National Institutes of Health Technology Assessment Conference," stated *"Available information indicates that BIA is not useful in measuring acute changes in body fat in individuals, although it can characterize longer term changes in groups of subjects. Measuring change by definition produces a larger error term by virtue of dependence on two (rather than one) imperfect measures, the error from which may be additive."* [82]

When considering the use of BIA, follow the advice from the Mayo Clinic: *"If you're concerned about your body fat percentage, skip the commercially available body fat analyzers...also called impedance meters... and ask your doctor about the use of more accurate measurement techniques."*[83]

Other Methods

More sophisticated methods for body measurements have been used in research studies. Quantification of body fat was needed for studies of the nature and treatment of obesity, and also for a variety of investigations that ranged from the assessment of nutritional status to the determination of the nature of the response of patients to a variety of diseases and metabolic disorders. Researchers used methods such as the determination of lean body mass by measurement of body potassium or body water, and the measurement of total body nitrogen by neutron activation[84].

Modern methods are available for use in clinical settings. For example, body fat can be estimated using cross-sectional imaging methods such as magnetic resonance imaging (MRI) and computerized tomography (CT). These scans can provide the most precise body composition measurements, especially for intra-abdominal fat measurement. They are expensive, however, and are usually not suggested solely for measuring body fat. Imaging tests such as ultrasound are not suggested solely for measuring body fat but could also be used.

Earlier we noted that BMI is not a measure of body fat. It was designed for population studies not for individuals. While body fat measurements techniques can in principle provide a better measure of percent body fat than BMI, they too are not suitable for individuals.

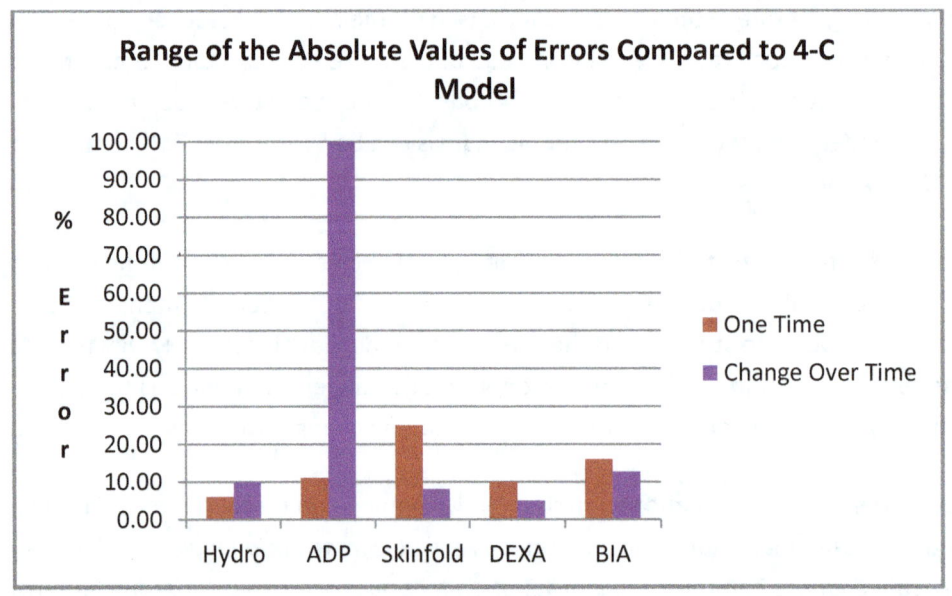

Due to their substantial errors of measurement none of the devices discussed here for measuring body fat and tracking – e.g. over 7 week intervals – an individual's body fat changes are adequate to warrant serious consideration. The errors of the measurement techniques can be greater than the changes that you are trying to measure. The chart above shows the range of absolute values (e.g. for plus or minus 4 the absolute value is 8) of the error for each of the techniques when compared to a four compartment model.

A person's needs could be better met using an accurate scale, a tape measure, and a mirror. Whether or not you choose to measure changes in weight or body fat, stay hydrated, get enough sleep, engage in daily exercise, and monitor the nutritional value of the food you eat.

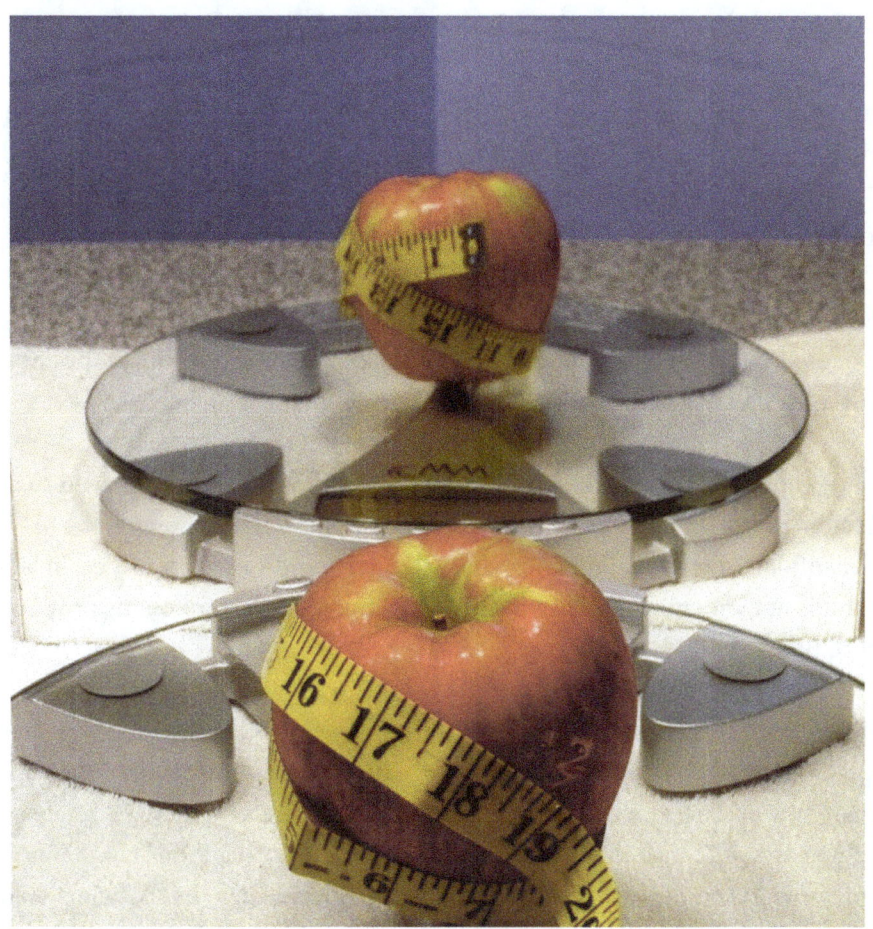

Nutrient Density

The Concept

The simplest concept of nutrient density is the ratio of nutrients to calories, n/c. As such, it is a measure of the nutrients provided per calorie of food. Nutrient density should be a more useful and analytically tractable ratio than BMI or percent body fat, which were designed to focus on the more elusive concept of healthy body composition. However, the implementation of the nutrient density concept is not straight forward.

For instance it does not account for the bioavailability of nutrients – the proportion of a nutrient that is absorbed from the diet and used for normal body functions. And there are practical problems when trying to use the ratio in a plug and chug manner. Like, for example, obtaining meaningful values in the numerator for phytochemicals. While the simple ratio is an elegant expression of an important concept, a more sophisticated mathematical approach is needed for the practical implementation the nutrient density concept.

Generally speaking, the nutrients include the macronutrients – carbohydrates, fats, and proteins – that provide calories and the micronutrients – vitamins and minerals – non-caloric substances that are indirectly involved in energy metabolism.

Additionally, water with zero calories is an essential nutrient[85]. It has numerous roles in the human body, which cannot produce enough water by metabolism or obtain enough water by food ingestion to fulfill its needs. We only get about 50% of the water we need from our food. Water acts as a building material, as a solvent, reaction medium, and reactant. It is a carrier for nutrients and waste products.

Water regulates the body temperature and serves as a lubricant and shock absorber[86]. Fruits and vegetables are generally high in water content, which provides volume and weight but not calories. Hence, they are low-energy-dense foods.

Phytochemicals are important non-nutritive, non-essential food components believed to be responsible for disease protection or prevention. Various phytochemicals have been shown to have anti-oxidant, anti-carcinogenic, anti-inflammatory, immunomodulatory, and anti-microbial effects in laboratory experiments. But it is not yet entirely clear whether consuming these compounds produces these or other effects in the body.

The nutrient density concept is useful for profiling foods and highlighting the most and least beneficial foods, but calculations based on a simple ratio of n/c are not sufficient measures for formulating a healthy meal or eating diet. The simple ratio does not provide for determining the relative quantities of various foods from across the range of nutrient density scores, including foods containing the many as yet unnamed and unmeasured beneficial phytochemicals, to include in a meal or diet. Hence, a more complete mathematical formulation is needed in place of a simple n/c ratio to create meaningful results.

Diet Formulation

The formulation of natural-ingredient diets is complicated by the fact that each ingredient contains many if not most nutrients, so that an adjustment in the amount of any ingredient produces changes in the concentrations of most nutrients in the final product. Hence it is not possible to predetermine the concentration of each nutrient; rather diets are formulated to contain minimal concentrations of particular nutrients

Diet formulation is a complex mathematical procedure. The human diet formulation problem can be restated as an optimization problem that <u>minimizes</u> the total energy content of the diet (that is called the "objective function") subject to various constraints, including satisfying recommended dietary allowances (RDA or some other set of reference values) for nutrients, allowing values for non-nutrients, and values for certain phytochemicals. The problem can be further constrained by limiting the food choices to plant based foods, excluding harmful foods or food products, and including provisions for exceptions, e.g. not all energy dense foods are nutrient poor (due to water content). It can even be constrained to limit or exclude the foods that don't taste good.

The human diet formulation problem is a type of optimization problem that can be solved with mathematical techniques know as linear and nonlinear programming. Many high school texts have sections on linear programming. The word programming here does not refer to a computer program (although linear programming problems are commonly solved using computer programs), it refers to planning to achieve an optimal mathematical result. A nonlinear program is similar to linear program but it includes at least one nonlinear function. However, non-linear programming is not straight forward from either mathematical or nutritional perspectives, and care needs to be taken to ensure that the data used and the models that are built up from the data are reasonable.

Historical Perspective on Linear Programming and Diet Formulation

Linear programming was developed as a mathematical discipline in the 1940, and the diet problem was among the first optimization problems that were studied. Solving the diet problem later became established as a popular exercise in college courses, particularly mathematics and operations research courses.

In 1950s, diet formulation was done by electromechanical machines and took one hour for the calculations. Following the advent of computers, computer solutions of diet optimization problems were used first for formulating animal diets, and much later for personalized diets in clinical and institutional practices [87].

Linear programming is frequently used by researchers to formulate diets based on estimates of nutrient density of foods in different food groups[88].

Solutions to the diet optimization problem using Microsoft Excel spreadsheet have been have been posted on the Web for many years. An ambitious reader with knowledge of elementary algebra and access to Excel or other spreadsheet software could create a spreadsheet to optimize their nutrient dense diets (see text box titled "A Special Project"). A desktop computer can solve such problems in milliseconds. A free, user-friendly diet analysis program, with a linear programming module, that minimizes cost can be examined online at the link furnished in endnote number 89 in the References [89].

> **A Special Project**
>
> The computer program technology is readily available to solve diet optimization problems, but high quality, user friendly, low cost software products are not yet available for fashioning daily meals optimized for nutrient density. If you would like to create such a program the link furnished in the endnote number 90 located in the References provides the code that can be used to perform the linear programming. You will have to build the interfaces that collect the input and display the results[90].

Implementing Nutrient Density

There have been numerous attempts to apply the nutrient density concept to profile or rate foods. Today there may be as many as ten competing systems, some of them depend upon proprietary algorithms. The nutrient content is computed in different ways by different systems.

One example is the naturally nutrient rich system (NNR). Nutrient density is defined as the ratio of the nutrient composition of a food to the nutrient requirements of the human. The NNR, in its simplest version is an average of per cent daily values (%DVs) for 14 key nutrients in 2000 calories of food. It is expressed with the following equation:

$$NNR = \sum \%DV_{2000 \text{ kcal}} / 14$$

The 14 nutrients are protein, thiamin, riboflavin, vitamin C, vitamin A, vitamin D, vitamin E, monounsaturated fat, calcium, potassium, iron, zinc, vitamin B_{12}, and folate. An updated description of the NNR score later added fiber and vitamin B_5 (pantothenic acid), for a total of 16 nutrients.

The FDA procedure for calculating %DV is to determine the ratio between the amount of the nutrient in a serving of food and the DV for the nutrient. That is, divide either the actual quantitative amount or the declared amount.

To calculate an NNR score for a serving of food, add up its percentage of daily values – the amount of each nutrient contained in a single serving as compared with the recommended daily intake of that nutrient – and divide it by the number of nutrients used (16 for the updated version).

The score ranges from two to 1,000. Any score over 100 is regarded as good and scores over 250 are considered to be excellent.

NNR can be used to assign nutrient density values to foods within and across food groups. However, the scores do not take into account the *bioavailability* of nutrients, e.g. calcium in milk is more bioavailable than is the calcium in spinach. A weighted NNR score would take bioavailability into account[91].

Another food rating approach is the **aggregate nutrient density index**, or ANDI, created by Dr. Joel Fuhrman. ANDI ranks the nutrient value of whole foods on the basis of how many nutrients they deliver to your body for each calorie consumed. ANDI scores are based on thirty-four nutritional parameters. Foods are ranked on a scale of 1-1000 with the most nutrient-dense cruciferous leafy green vegetables scoring 1000. ANDI rankings (and other rankings) may underestimate the healthful properties of colorful, natural, plant foods because phytochemicals are largely unnamed and unmeasured. ANDI highly ranks green vegetables, especially compared to processed foods and animal products.

ANDI Nutrient Scoring Method

To determine the ANDI scores, an equal-calorie serving of each food was evaluated.

The following nutrients were included in the evaluation: fiber, calcium, iron, magnesium, phosphorus, potassium, zinc, copper, manganese, selenium, vitamin A, beta carotene, alpha carotene, lycopene, lutein and zeaxanthin, vitamin E, vitamin C, thiamin, riboflavin, niacin, pantothenic acid, vitamin B_6, folate, vitamin B_{12}, choline, vitamin K, phytosterols, glucosinolates, angiogenesis inhibitors, organosulfides, aromatase inhibitors, resistant starch, resveratrol plus the ORAC score.

ORAC (Oxygen Radical Absorbance Capacity) is a measure of the antioxidant or radical scavenging capacity of a food. For consistency, nutrient quantities were converted from their typical measurement conventions (mg, mcg, IU) to a percentage of their Dietary Reference Intake (DRI). For nutrients that have no DRI, goals were established based on available research and current understanding of the benefits of these factors. To make it easier to compare foods, the raw point totals were converted (multiplied by the same number) so that the highest ranking foods (leafy green vegetables) received a score of 1000, and the other foods received lower scores accordingly[92].

The ANDI scoring method is presented in more detail in the text box. Additional information is included in the Appendix concerning the phytosterols, glucosinolates, angiogenesis inhibitors, organosulfides, aromatase inhibitors, resistant starch, resveratrol, and ORAC score. Phytochemicals are discussed in Chapter Five.

Dr. Fuhrman advises people to consume mostly foods that have an ANDI score greater than 100, but he also recommends eating an adequate assortment of lower ranked plant foods to obtain the full range of human requirements. He suggests eating greens, beans, onions, mushrooms, berries, and seeds every day because of their powerful anti-cancer and anti-fat storage effects. And he cautions that nutrient density scoring is not the only factor that determines good health. *"For example, if we only ate foods with a high nutrient density score our diet would be too low in fat."* The ANDI scores are available at Dr. Fuhrman's website and Whole Foods Market's websites.

The nutrient content is computed in yet another food rating approach: The aforementioned NNR equation was refined to create a scoring system to estimate the **nutritional adequacy** of vegetables and fruits, on a per weight, per calorie, and per unit cost basis. Subsequently, the NNR equation was adopted to calculate nutrient density as the method used to define *"powerhouse fruits and vegetables"* – foods most strongly associated with reduced chronic disease risk[93].

In this method the numerator is a nutrient adequacy score calculated as the mean of percent daily values (DVs) for the qualifying nutrients based on a 2,000 kcal/day diet per 100 grams of food. The scores were weighted using available data based on the bioavailability of the nutrients:

$$\text{Nutrient adequacy score} = (\Sigma\ [\text{nutrient}_i \times \text{bioavailability}_i]/DV_i] \times 100)/17$$

Because some foods are excellent sources of a particular nutrient but contain few other nutrients, percent DVs were capped at 100 so that any one nutrient would not contribute unduly to the total score. The denominator is the energy density of the food (kilocalories per 100 g):

$$\text{Nutrient density score (expressed per 100 kcal)} = (\text{nutrient adequacy score}/\text{energy density}) \times 100$$

The score represents the mean of percent DVs per 100 kcal of food. Nutrient-dense foods (defined as those with scores ≥10) were classified as powerhouse fruits and vegetables. The authored noted that *"because it was not possible to include phytochemical data in the calculation of nutrient density scores, the scores do not reflect all of the constituents that may confer health benefits."*

Using this method, the score for watercress is 100, while that for kale is 49.07[94].

Nutrient density scores reported for the same substances using different methods of calculation can vary substantially. For example watercress and kale scored at 1000 on a 1000 point scoring system under ANDI, compared to 100 for watercress and only 49.07 for kale on the 100 point scoring system discussed above.

Additional methods to implement the nutrient density concept can be expected to be developed. There are still challenges associated with the implementation of the nutrient density concept. However, it is by far the most reliable single indicator of the nutrient content of foods. If you choose foods that are both high in nutrient density and low in energy density, you are more likely to consume more nutrients and less calories.

When considering the use of nutrient density models or systems, try to determine how the nutritional values are derived, and the underlying assumptions. Look for credible reviews that identify limitations of the model or system. Try to avoid models and systems based on proprietary, "black-box," algorithms. They are not subject to independent reviews and validation.

Don't accept dogma and risk compromising a healthy diet. A diet of healthful eating is important for disease prevention, maintenance of a healthy weight, quality of life, and longevity. A healthy diet will give you vitality and energy for life.

Food for Thought

1. Several anthropometric surrogate markers such as the body adiposity index (BAI), the body mass index (BMI), waist-to-hip ratio (WHR) and waist-to-height ratio (WHtR) have been discussed for use in clinical practice. Is there any evidence that each adds to the predictive power of the others, and a combination of two or more indexes are superior to the separate indicators in identifying risk of disorders and disease risks?

2. Obesity is known to be associated with metabolic disturbances including insulin resistance and inflammation. However, there are obese subjects who have normal metabolic profiles, and do not seem to be at an increased risk for metabolic complications of obesity.

These individuals are described as metabolically healthy but obese (MHO), or as having uncomplicated obesity, or metabolically benign obesity. Despite having excessive body fat, people who are metabolically healthy but obese have favorable metabolic profiles, characterized by remarkably high insulin sensitivity, no sign of hypertension, and normal lipid, inflammation, and hormonal profiles (low triglycerides and C-reactive protein concentrations and high HDL cholesterol and adiponectin concentrations)[95].

Importantly, individuals with MHO do not significantly improve their cardio-metabolic risk upon weight loss interventions and therefore may not benefit to the same extent as obese patients with metabolic comorbidities from early lifestyle, bariatric surgery, or pharmacological interventions. Are MHO individuals really healthy?[96]

3. Screening and retention of military recruits, policemen, firemen, and other workers in whom high fitness levels are required are often based on BMI standards and in some cases on a second-tier body fat evaluation. A person with a BMI equal to 40 or more would be classified as morbidly obese. The 2014 World's Strongest Man winner Žydrūnas Savickas had a BMI of 46.9 Is BMI profiling a reasonable measure of fitness?

4. It is unclear whether increased retroperitoneal fat is a cause or the result of mechanisms that increase blood pressure associated with obesity. For obese people with hypertension, which organs in the retroperitoneal area would you expect to be surrounded by fat? [97]

5. **Explain why** watercress and kale each scored at 1000 on a 1000 point scoring system under ANDI, but using the Powerhouse Fruits and Vegetables system watercress scored 100 but the score for kale was only 49.07 on the 100 point scoring system.

Chapter Three: Food Labels

If you are what you eat and you don't know what you're eating, do you know what you are? – Vulnerable!

When foraging for healthy foods it is often necessary to obtain accurate information about the nutrient and energy content of food products from various sources. That can be a challenging task.

Health conscious eaters tend to be avid label readers. Most packaged foods are required by law to carry nutrition labeling. This labeling is voluntary for many raw foods, such as fruits, vegetables, and fish. The Food and Drug Administration (FDA) encourages stores that sell raw foods to display or distribute, near these foods, nutrition information to shoppers. To make it easy for retailers, FDA has created colorful posters that can be downloaded and printed from its Web site. The posters show nutrition information for the 20 most frequently consumed raw fruits, vegetables, and fish in the United States. The posters can been viewed by using the link in endnote number 98 that is the provided in the References[98].

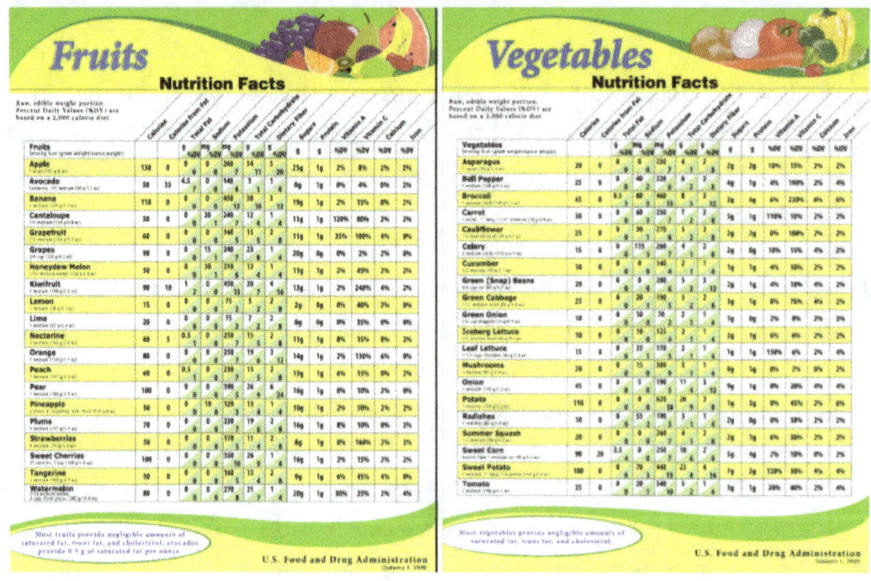

Customers are encouraged to ask at the store for the nutrition information for those raw foods if it is not displayed. FDA also encourages consumers to request nutrition information in full-service or fast-food restaurants.

Under current federal regulations, providing nutrition information for restaurant food is voluntary unless a nutrient content claim or a health claim is made for a menu item or meal. For example, a nutrient content claim might be *"low in fat,"* and a health claim might be *"heart healthy."* If such claims are made, the restaurant is required to give customers the appropriate nutrition information for these items when requested. This information does not have to be on the menu or on a menu board that's clearly visible to the consumer. The restaurant has the option of offering this information in various ways, such as in a brochure. Some states, localities, and large restaurant chains were already doing their own forms of menu labeling.

FDA proposed new regulations that required calorie information on restaurant menus and menu boards by December 1, 2015 and on vending machines by December 1, 2016. However, FDA later extended the compliance date for an additional year (December 1, 2016) in response to pressure from chain restaurants, pizza parlors and movie theaters. The pizza industry lobby argued that the calorie display would be too labor-intensive and costly[99].

Many food service establishments have nutrition information for their offerings and can be expected to provide the information on the Internet or to customers who request it.

FDA regulations require that most nutrients must be declared on the Nutrition Facts Label as *"percent Daily Value"* (%DV), which tells the percent of the recommended daily intake in a serving of that product and is supposed to help the consumer to create a balanced diet. The %DV was designed by the FDA to allow consumers to see at a glance if a product has a high or low amount of a nutrient. **The rule of thumb is 20% DV or more is high and 5% DV or less is low.** The %DV is calculated from the DVs listed for food components on the FDA website. The link for that website page is provided at endnote number 100 in the References[100].

The term "organic" is not defined by law or regulations FDA enforces. Food labeled "organic" must meet the standards set by the Department of Agriculture (USDA). Organic food differs from conventionally produced food in the way it is grown or produced. But USDA makes no claims that organically produced food is safer or more nutritious than conventionally produced food. According to USDA rules, if 95 percent of a product is made up of organic ingredients, it can be called organic. But the organic food could include approved non-organic additives and could be exposed to approved chemicals that are supposedly safe for humans. The non-organic 5 percent could be sprayed with herbicides and pesticides. If it's 70 percent organic, the label can read *"made with organic ingredients."*

The USDA has recently proposed to amend the origin of livestock requirements for dairy animals under the USDA organic regulations. The intent of the proposed new rule is to prevent the practice of raising calves on medicated milk replacer that includes antibiotics and, after weaning, feeding them GMO grains and hay treated with toxic pesticides, instead of raising the calves on organic milk. But critics argue that a loophole in the proposed rule will allow flagrant abuses to keep occurring. They point out that some industrial scale organic dairies have been flouting this rule for years by continuously purchasing conventional replacement heifers (young cows) that have been transitioned to organic. They want the a rule that ensures that *"no young transitioned heifers, who have never been milked, could qualify to be sold as 'organic' "* [101].

The USDA also publishes guidance for the limits on consumption of empty calories. Empty calories are defined as calories from solid fats or added sugars that contain few or no nutrients[102].

Readers are encouraged to visit the FDA webpage titled "How to Understand and Use the Nutrition Facts Label" for a detailed presentation on understanding current food labels[103].

Original Label

Nutrition Facts	
Serving Size 2/3 cup (55g)	
Servings Per Container About 8	
Amount Per Serving	
Calories 230	Calories from Fat 72
	% Daily Value*
Total Fat 8g	12%
Saturated Fat 1g	5%
Trans Fat 0g	
Cholesterol 0mg	0%
Sodium 160mg	7%
Total Carbohydrate 37g	12%
Dietary Fiber 4g	16%
Sugars 1g	
Protein 3g	
Vitamin A	10%
Vitamin C	8%
Calcium	20%
Iron	45%

* Percent Daily Values are based on a 2,000 calorie diet. Your daily value may be higher or lower depending on your calorie needs.

	Calories:	2,000	2,500
Total Fat	Less than	65g	80g
Sat Fat	Less than	20g	25g
Cholesterol	Less than	300mg	300mg
Sodium	Less than	2,400mg	2,400mg
Total Carbohydrate		300g	375g
Dietary Fiber		25g	30g

Proposed Label

Nutrition Facts	
8 servings per container	
Serving size	2/3 cup (55g)
Amount per 2/3 cup	
Calories	**230**
% DV*	
12%	**Total Fat** 8g
5%	Saturated Fat 1g
	Trans Fat 0g
0%	**Cholesterol** 0mg
7%	**Sodium** 160mg
12%	**Total Carbs** 37g
14%	Dietary Fiber 4g
	Sugars 1g
	Added Sugars 0g
	Protein 3g
10%	Vitamin D 2mcg
20%	Calcium 260mg
45%	Iron 8mg
5%	Potassium 235mg

* Footnote on Daily Values (DV) and calories reference to be inserted here.

The FDA's proposed update of the twenty years old Nutrition Facts label, currently found on most food packages in the United States, is presented on FDA's webpage[104]. The updated version is also controversial. For example, its serving sizes are not consistent with the HHS/USDA Dietary Guidelines for Americans. The proposed serving sizes could encourage overeating by listing single serving size of an entire pint of ice cream or a 20 ounce bottle of soda. Additionally, the labels still rely on a 2,000-kcal diet to derive the percent Daily Values[105]. Those serving sizes may be typical of consumption patterns of the more than two thirds of Americans who are overweight and obese[106].

Food labels don't list a food's **glycemic index** score and very few companies are including the information on product labels. The glycemic index[107], which is discussed in the next chapter, is a measure of how a carbohydrate containing food raises blood glucose. It is a ranking of carbohydrates on a scale from 0 to 100.

You may also want to know the **glycemic load**, a numerical value that indicates the change in blood glucose levels when you eat a typical serving of the food. A food's glycemic load is determined by multiplying its glycemic index by the amount of carbohydrate in grams the food contains and dividing by 100. **In general, a glycemic load of 20 or more is high, 11 to 19 is medium, and 10 or under is low.** Thus glycemic load is a means of capturing both the quality and quantity of dietary carbohydrates. **Dietary glycemic load** is the sum of the glycemic loads for all foods consumed in the diet.

Note that the glycemic index of particular foods depends on several factors, including its processing or how it's cooked. The glycemic index can be a useful indicator to guide food choice if for example bread with a high GI is replaced on a slice-for-slice basis with a lower GI bread, thereby achieving a lower GL.

In the absence of GI and GL information the consumer has to examine the products and ask key questions. To guess how much the food will raise a person's blood glucose level after eating it you need to know the composition of the food. For example, watermelon has a high GI, but a single serving is mostly water with a small amount of carbohydrates. Therefore, the GL of watermelon is relatively low. In the case of bread, question what grain was used to make it. Is the grain whole, coarsely ground, finely ground, milled and refined? Knowing that processing most grains increases their glycemic index, might help you make an educated guess about an unlabeled product.

Harvard School of Public Health recommends using an index for breads and cereals, which is the ratio of the number of grams per serving of carbohydrates to the number of grams of fiber per serving, symbolically **C/F**. Scores of 5 and under for cereals and 10 and under for breads are considered to be good sources of carbohydrates[108]. The C/F ratio is the subject of considerable interest in research studies.

Researchers recently showed that snack food (potato chips) intake in satiated rats is triggered by an optimal fat/carbohydrate ratio. They tested the then prevailing hypothesis that the food's energy density may be the crucial factor that triggers food intake beyond satiety resulting in elevated weight and, eventually, in obesity. Behavioral preference tests were conducted to investigate the intake of foods with different fat/carbohydrate contents and MRI measurements were performed to investigate the modulation of whole brain activity induced in rats.

The study concluded from behavioral data that the ratio of fat and carbohydrates, but not the absolute energy density, is the major determinant of the palatability and intake of snack food during short-term two-choice preference tests in rats. From the imaging approach, it was concluded that the energy density alone is only a moderate determinant of the rewarding properties of snack food. However the authors stated, *"Although the ratio of fat and carbohydrates of potato chips seems to be highly attractive, it can be hypothesized that other molecular determinants [emphasis added] exist in this snack food, which modulate the activity of brain circuits, particularly the reward system, even stronger and lead to increased food seeking behavior."*[109]

Product labels frequently contain long lists of food additives, many of them unfamiliar, and some that you will want to avoid in any food you consume may be masked by food additive numbers or vague but legal terms. Additives are discussed in the next chapter. The References contain links to articles that discuss deceptive labeling practices, which are also discussed below. It is important to read and understand what the **listed ingredients** are and how they may affect you.

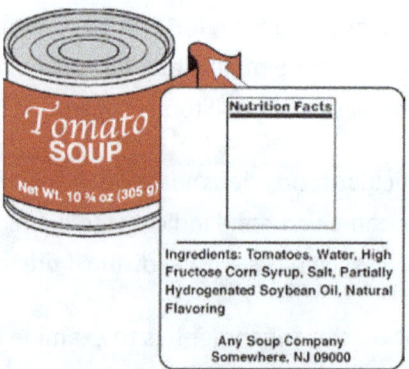

For example, ingredients are ordered by volume, so the higher up on the list an ingredient is, the more of it a product contains. Food manufacturers are required to label food products that are made with an ingredient that is a major food allergen in one of the following two ways:

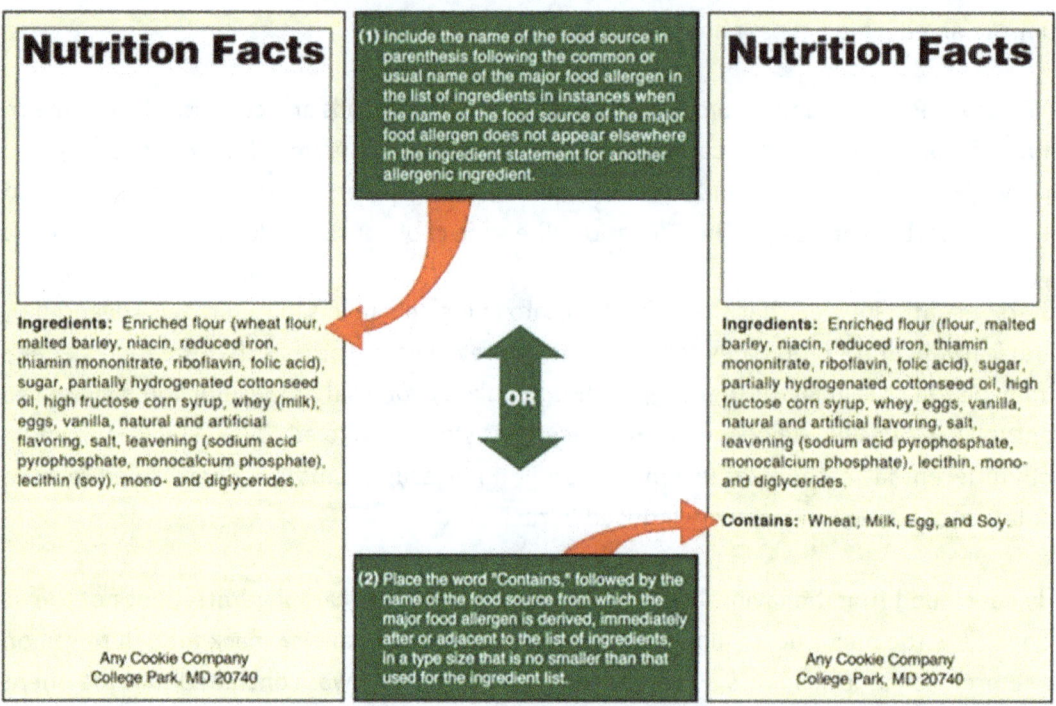

Ingredients lists on food products are supposed to inform consumers about the contents of the products. Unfortunately, ingredients lists are often used by food manufacturers to deceive consumers by exploiting the loopholes in the government's lax labeling regulations. That has resulted in the publication of helpful tips and strategies for example, *"Sometimes, manufacturers split up sugar into dextrose, high-fructose corn syrup, cane crystals and so on, so none of them are the first ingredient, even though if you added*

them up, they would be," explains Walter Willett, MD. "You might consider avoiding any product if there is sugar in more than one form." [110]

Another example: *"When the Nutrition Facts label says a food contains "0 g" of trans fat, but includes "partially hydrogenated oil" in the ingredient list, it means the food contains trans fat, but less than 0.5 grams of trans fat per serving. So, if you eat more than one serving, you could quickly reach your daily limit of trans fat."*[111]

Food labels may not provide sufficient information for a comprehensive analysis. However, careful use of the Nutrition Facts labels, augmented by detailed nutrient information that can be found on the Web should provide sufficient information about the nutrients and caloric values in your foods to formulate healthful diets.

Food for Thought

1. The %DV was designed by the FDA to allow consumers to see at a glance if a product has a high or low amount of a nutrient. The rule of thumb is **20% DV or more is high and 5% DV or less is low**. Is the rule of thumb printed on product labels? Where can consumers find the rule thumb?

2. Carbohydrates have 4 calories per gram and fat has 9 calories per gram. Would you expect that a reduction of dietary fat compared to carbohydrates would be an effective weight loss strategy or a strategy focused on whole foods, portion size, and healthy eating patterns?

3. A clever person posted examples of what the ingredient labels might look like for natural whole foods[112]. In the figures below which E number designates the anthocynanins?

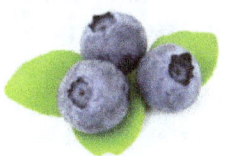
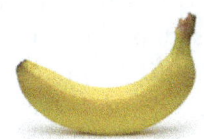

Chapter Four: Don't Eat *That*!

"Snow White longed for the beautiful apple, and when she saw that the peddler woman was eating part of it she could no longer resist, and she stuck her hand out and took the poisoned half. She barely had a bite in her mouth when she fell to the ground dead."

Now that we know how to determine the nutrient and energy values of foods, we turn to addressing the questions, "What are the healthful foods? And, "What foods should we limit or avoid?" In this chapter you will discover how to determine what foods to limit or avoid. Let's begin with the poor food choices, the foods to avoid, before discussing the substances that you should limit. At the top of the list are the so-called junk foods and comfort food. Many of them are delicious, conveniently available, frequently used for socialization, self-medication, and even fun to eat. And since no two tastes are exactly alike, comfort foods are different for different people.

Nutrient Profiling

Television advertising is known to be an important influence on children's preferences for food and drinks and most of the food products promoted have an undesirable nutritional profile. Nutrient profile models classify or rank foods according to their nutritional composition for reasons related to prevention of disease and promotion of health.

Many nutrient profile models have been developed by academics, health charities, national governments and the food industry, some of which have been designed to regulate the broadcast advertising of foods.

Nutrient profile models can be used to identifying those foods that should (or should not) be advertised to children. In 2010 the World Health Assembly passed a resolution endorsing WHO recommendations to *"reduce both the exposure of children to, and power of, marketing of foods high in saturated fats, trans-fatty acids, free sugars or salt,"* and the resolution urged member states to implement the recommendations[113].

Bagels, bacon, baked ziti, barbecued meats, beef stew, biscuits, brownies, cakes, cheese, cheeseburgers, chicken pot pie, chicken tetrazzini, chicken fried steak, chili (beef, chicken, turkey), chips, chocolate pudding, cinnamon rolls, cobblers, cookies, corn bread, crackers, donuts, dumplings, French fries, French onion soup, French toast, fried chicken, grilled cheese, hamburgers, hot dogs, ice cream, lasagna, luncheon meats, mac and cheese, mashed potatoes with gravy, meatloaf, muffins, pies, pizza, pork chops, pot roast, red meat, roast beef, sausage, smoked meat, sodas, spaghetti and meatballs, strawberry shortcake, tacos, tuna melts, waffles, and frozen yogurt are comfort foods-- to name a few.

Few people would quit eating junk foods and comfort foods without alternatives that are at least as delicious, conveniently available, valuable for social connectivity, useful for self-medication, and even fun. However, it is worthwhile taking the time to read food labels, inquire about the contents, and consider some of the potential consequences of continuing to eat junk foods, comfort foods, and other food products. Knowing what is in them, how they are prepared, and their caloric contents might convince you to try to find other alternatives. Keep in mind that the risks associated with unhealthful foods may vary depending on your genetics and you health status.

Macronutrients

Fats are twice as energy rich as proteins and carbohydrates. Extra fat is stored by the body and it is used as fuel after carbohydrates are no longer available. Fat is an essential nutrient. Too little of too much fat will result in poor health.

Trans fats (or trans fatty acids) are not naturally occurring in humans. The artificial trans fats are created in an industrial process that adds hydrogen to liquid vegetable oils to make them more solid. Trans fats are found in many of the foods listed above, including but not limited to biscuits, cakes, cinnamon rolls, cookies, crackers, frozen pies, pizza, coffee creamers, fast food, microwave popcorn, vegetable shortenings and stick margarines.

Eating foods containing trans fat significantly increases your risk of heart disease because it raises LDL cholesterol and lowers HDL cholesterol. Trans fat is put into food by adding partially hydrogenated vegetable oil. The solidified vegetable oils give products a longer shelf life, and the oils also last longer in deep fryers. You can avoid trans fats by reading food labels and finding out what kind of oils your restaurants use. Note that product labels that list zero grams of trans fats might still have some amount of partially hydrogenated vegetable oil listed elsewhere on the label. Medical experts caution that even the smallest amounts of trans fats are not acceptable[114].

Like trans fats, saturated fats are solid at room temperature. This type of fat comes mainly from animal sources of food, such as red meat, poultry and full-fat dairy products like cheese. Saturated fat raises total blood cholesterol levels and LDL cholesterol levels, which prompts blockages to form in arteries in the heart and elsewhere in the body. Limiting saturated fat consumption has been a longstanding dietary recommendation to reduce risk of cardiovascular disease and type 2 diabetes. However, according to the Harvard Medical School:

"A handful of recent reports have muddied the link between saturated fat and heart disease. One meta-analysis of 21 studies said that there was not enough evidence to conclude that saturated fat increases the risk of heart disease, but that replacing saturated fat with polyunsaturated fat may indeed reduce risk of heart disease." [115]

"Two other major studies narrowed the prescription slightly, concluding that replacing saturated fat with polyunsaturated fats like vegetable oils or high-fiber carbohydrates is the best bet for reducing the risk of heart disease, but replacing saturated fat with highly processed carbohydrates could do the opposite." [116]

The Scientific Report of the 2015 Dietary Guidelines Advisory Committee to the Secretaries of the U.S. Departments of Health and Human Services and Agriculture concluded that sources of saturated fat should be replaced with unsaturated fat, particularly polyunsaturated fatty acids[117].

Carbohydrates are the source of glucose which is the most essential source of energy in the body. Just like other cells brain cells use glucose to power cellular activity, but the brain works entirely on glucose. Too little of too much carbohydrates will result in poor health.

Foods that have similar carbohydrate content can differ in the amount they raise blood glucose. Avoid eating a lot of high-glycemic-index foods, which are rapidly digested and absorbed or transformed metabolically into glucose. High GI foods such as refined grain products or potatoes can have GI values that exceed table sugar (GI=58,GL=6) by up to fifty percent. The powerful spikes in blood sugar can lead to increased risk for type 2 diabetes, heart disease, and being overweight. And the Nutrition Source at Harvard reports that there is preliminary work linking high GI diets to age-related macular degeneration, ovulatory infertility, and colorectal cancer.

Tropical fruits, carrots and beets are included among foods that have a high glycemic index. Most of these foods have a low glycemic load, so the amount of sugar provided in an average serving is unlikely to significantly increase blood sugar[118]. Aim to lower your dietary glycemic load. A list of the GI and glycemic loads for more than 100 foods can be found at the website link number 119 in the References[119].

Proteins are the last macronutrient to be used as a source of energy. The muscles in the body are devoured to provide energy during starvation. Dietary protein is used to build new cells, maintain tissues, and synthesize new proteins, like enzymes, to perform vital functions. Too little of too much protein will result in poor health.

The American Institute for Cancer Research cautions that eating too much of any red meat – more than 18 ounces cooked, weekly – increases risk for colorectal cancer. Red meats that are processed red meats – such as bacon, hot dogs, and sausage – are also available in leaner forms, yet even small amounts of these meats, eaten regularly, lead to higher risk for colorectal cancer – which is a cancer that starts either in the colon or rectum. Processed meats are also consistently linked to increased risk of heart disease and type 2 diabetes. Research also suggests that gut bacteria may convert compounds in red meat to substances that promote atherosclerosis and/or cause less healthful types of bacteria in the intestinal tract to flourish[120].

In October 2015, after reviewing the accumulated scientific literature, a Working Group of 22 experts from 10 countries convened by WHO's International Agency for Research on Cancer (IARC) classified the consumption of red meat as *"probably carcinogenic to humans (Group 2A), based on limited evidence that the consumption of red meat causes cancer in humans and strong mechanistic evidence supporting a carcinogenic effect. This association was observed mainly for colorectal cancer, but associations were also seen for pancreatic cancer and prostate cancer….Processed meat was classified as carcinogenic to humans*

(Group 1), based on sufficient evidence in humans that the consumption of processed meat causes colorectal cancer."[121]

IARC Classification

IARC classifies carcinogens in five categories ranging from carcinogenic to humans (Group 1) to probably not carcinogenic to humans (Group 4). The classification indicates the weight of the evidence as to whether an agent is capable of causing cancer (technically called "hazard"), but it does not measure the likelihood that cancer will occur (technically called "risk") as a result of exposure to the agent.

Group 1: The agent is carcinogenic to humans. This category is used when there is sufficient evidence of carcinogenicity in humans.

Group 2A: The agent is probably carcinogenic to humans. This category is used when there is limited evidence of carcinogenicity in humans and sufficient evidence of carcinogenicity in experimental animals.

Food preparation can be very important. According to the FDA, high temperature cooking, such as frying, roasting, or baking, is most likely to cause the formation of acrylamide, a chemical that forms from sugars and an amino acid (asparagine) that are naturally present in food. Acrylamide is a human health concern. In large doses, this chemical has caused cancer in laboratory animals.

Acrylamide is found mainly in foods made from plants, such as potato products, grain products, or coffee. Frying leads to highest acrylamide formation followed by roasting, then by baking. The darker the potato, the more acrylamide. Similarly, it is advisable to toast bread to a light brown color and avoid very brown areas[122].

Finally, it is generally accepted that adding fat and protein to carbohydrate reduces blood glucose compared with carbohydrate alone. This suggests that replacing some carbohydrate content with healthy dietary fats and protein could therefore result in steadier overall levels of blood sugar and yield a better overall blood sugar response.

Vitamins and Minerals Supplements

FDA regulates dietary supplements under a different set of regulations than those covering *"conventional"* foods and drug products. A dietary supplement is a product taken by mouth that contains a *"dietary ingredient"* intended to supplement the diet. The *"dietary ingredients"* in these products may include: vitamins, minerals, herbs or other botanicals, amino acids, and substances such as enzymes, organ tissues, glandulars, and metabolites. In this section we will briefly discuss vitamin and mineral supplements.

Because supplements are not regulated as conventional foods and drug products by the FDA, **consumers cannot rely entirely on the information printed on their labels to be sure of their safety and efficacy.** Supplemental vitamins and minerals can interact in ways that can counteract their intended purposes and also affect the absorption and effectiveness of medications. They can even create faulty results on medical lab tests. Therefore it is important to review reliable information about their safety and interactions before you purchase supplements. You should do your home work. Ask your pharmacist. Check the facts. There are *"interactions checkers"* available on the Web. You need especially to be wary about supplement interactions and overdoses.

It is dangerous to consume too much of anything, even water. **Eating fortified foods while also taking supplements can cause a person's diet to exceed safe upper levels.** Here we will briefly discuss the risks associated with the <u>excess consumption</u> of some important vitamins and minerals.

Vitamins and minerals are nutrients required in very small amounts for essential metabolic reactions in the body. High doses of vitamins are unnecessary and can be risky. The Tolerable Upper Intake Levels (UL) has been established by the National Academy of Sciences, Institute of Medicine for some vitamins and minerals. ULs can be found at the website link number 123 in the References[123].

The UL represents the highest average daily intake level that is likely to pose no risk of adverse health effects to almost all individuals in the general population. The UL includes how much of a nutrient you get from both food and supplements. Read carefully the Supplement Labels and try to stay under the UL.

Vitamin Supplements

There is nothing simple about vitamins. A *"vitamin"* frequently refers to more than one chemical compound, for example there are three active forms of vitamin A in the human body – retinol, retinal, and retinoic acid. Additionally, there are two different types of vitamin A, preformed vitamin A found in animal products and provitamin A carotenoids found in plant-based products. Beta-carotene is the most common type of provitamin A.

Vitamin A, a fat soluble vitamin, is predominately stored in the liver. At high doses it is toxic to the liver. Hypervitaminosis A it caused by overconsumption of preformed vitamin A, not carotenoids. The UL does not apply to vitamin A derived from carotenoids. Signs of acute vitamin A toxicity are nausea, headache, fatigue, loss of appetite, dizziness, dry skin, and cerebral edema. Symptoms of chronic toxicity include anemia, anorexia, headache, weight loss, bone and joint pain, dry itchy skin, cerebral edema, enlarged liver, and enlarged spleen. Severe cases can end in liver damage, hemorrhage, coma and death.

Ingesting too much preformed vitamin A during early pregnancy can cause severe developmental abnormalities in the fetus. But, according to the Linus Pauling Institute there is no evidence that consumption of vitamin A from beta carotene might increase the risk of birth defects[124]. High potency vitamin A supplements should not be used without medical supervision due to the risk of toxicity.

The B vitamins are water soluble, they do not require fat to be absorbed, and they do not accumulate in the body. The B vitamins include: B_1 (thiamine), B_2 (riboflavin), B_3 (niacin), B_5 (pantothenic acid), B_6, B_7 (biotin), B_{12}, and Folic acid. There are no vitamins named B_4, B_8, B_{10}, and B_{11} because those substances were originally mistakenly thought to be essential nutrients.

Vitamin B_3 has two other forms in addition to niacin. A common minor side effect of niacin is a flushing reaction. This might cause burning, tingling, itching, and redness of the face, arms, and chest, as well as headaches. Other minor side effects of niacin and niacinamide are stomach upset, intestinal gas, dizziness, pain in the mouth, and additional problems.

Niacin overdose signs and symptoms include severe skin flushing combined with dizziness, rapid heartbeat, itching, nausea and vomiting, abdominal pain, diarrhea, and gout. High doses and certain formulations of niacin have been linked to acute liver injury which can be severe as well as fatal. Significant hepatotoxicity is particularly common with high doses of sustained release niacin[125].

Pyridoxine is the supplemental form of vitamin B_6. Very high doses causes neuropathy, the disease or dysfunction of one or more peripheral nerves. Large daily doses of the vitamin B_6 have been associated with neurological problems, such as numbness in the hands and feet (peripheral neuropathy), and walking may become unstable and labored[126].

Folate is a general term for a group of water soluble B-vitamins, and is also known as B_9. Folic acid refers to the oxidized synthetic compound used in dietary supplements and food fortification. **Deficiencies of either folate or vitamin B_{12} can cause red blood cells to enlarge, a condition known as megaloblastic anemia.** Taking synthetic folic acid alone can mask symptoms of B_{12} deficiency, since folic acid can cause the blood cells affected by B_{12} deficiency to return to normal. The presence of enlarged blood cells is used to determine vitamin B_{12} status, despite the fact that deficiency and associated symptoms can occur below the level at which blood cells are affected. The result, regardless of the presence of enlarged blood cells, is that a potentially serious B_{12} deficiency may remain undiagnosed **and could result in irreversible nerve damage.** High serum folate might also exacerbate the anemia and worsen cognitive symptoms of the deficiency.

According to Fuhrman, many Americans, through multivitamin use and consumption of fortified foods, are taking in excessive amounts of folic acid, which is not modified to folate by intestinal cells, and thus they may have unmodified folic acid circulating in their blood which could contribute to the cancer-promoting effects[127].

Vitamin C (aka ascorbic acid) is water soluble. Vitamin C is an anti-oxidant. Excess vitamin C can cause diarrhea, nausea, vomiting, heartburn, abdominal bloating and cramps, headache, insomnia, and kidney stones[128].

Vitamin D is fat soluble. It is important for bone health. It aids in calcium absorption, but too much can lead to an overabundance of calcium in the blood, which could cause poor appetite, nausea, vomiting, weakness, and frequent urination. Excessive vitamin D, might cause kidney damage[129].

Vitamin E is a fat-soluble anti-oxidant. Excess levels of vitamin E may increase the risk of hemorrhaging. Taking very high doses may interfere with the body's ability to clot blood, posing a risk to people taking prescribed blood thinners or aspirin[130].

Vitamin K is fat soluble. It is essential for the functions of several proteins including, but not limited to, their role in blood clotting. No toxic level has been set for vitamin K_1 (phytonadione) and K_2 (menaquinone). Consuming excessive vitamin K_3 (menadione) might lead to permanent damage to cell membranes. When given to infants by injection, K_3 has induced liver toxicity, jaundice, and hemolytic anemia. Excess vitamin K can lessen or reverse the effect of blood thinner medicines and prevent normal blood clotting[131].

Mineral Supplements

Minerals are stored throughout the body and little amounts are excreted, so the risk of toxicity from consuming excess minerals is high. Important bioactive minerals include calcium, chromium, copper, fluoride, iodine, iron, magnesium, manganese, molybdenum, phosphorus, potassium, selenium, sodium, and zinc. The published value for the ULs, the tolerable upper intake levels, can be found at the link in number 132 in the References[132].

Some concerns regarding the dangers associated with excessive consumption of important minerals are briefly discussed below.

Excess Calcium

Taking too many calcium supplements causes hypercalcemia, the medical term for too much calcium in the blood. This condition is called *"milk-alkali syndrome,"* the name originally used to refer to hypercalcemia that was the result of prescribing milk and sodium bicarbonate for the treatment of peptic ulcers. The original milk-alkali syndrome became a rarity with the advent of modern ulcer therapy.

Today, hypercalcemia is better described as the calcium-alkali syndrome and the common sources of the calcium and alkali are antacids and supplements taken to prevent osteoporosis. Mild hypercalcemia may result in loss of appetite, nausea, vomiting, constipation, abdominal pain, fatigue, frequent urination, and hypertension. More severe hypercalcemia may result in confusion, delirium, coma, and if not treated, death. A high level of vitamin D in the body, such as from taking supplements, can worsen milk-alkali syndrome [133].

Excess Iron

Dietary iron occurs in two forms, heme iron and nonheme iron. Plants and iron-fortified foods contain nonheme iron. Meats, seafood, and poultry contain both heme and nonheme iron. Individuals who are not at risk of iron deficiency should not take iron supplements without a medical evaluation[134].

Taking iron from supplements or medicines can lead to gastric upset, constipation, nausea, abdominal pain, vomiting, and faintness, especially if food is not taken at the same time. Larger doses of elemental iron can reduce zinc absorption and plasma zinc concentrations. In severe cases overdoses of iron can lead to multisystem organ failure, coma, convulsions, and death[135].

Excess Magnesium

The initial symptom of excess magnesium from dietary supplements is diarrhea that can be accompanied by nausea and abdominal cramping. Very large doses of magnesium in laxatives and antacids have been associated with magnesium toxicity, which can include hypotension, nausea, vomiting, facial flushing, retention of urine, intestinal blockage (ileus), depression and lethargy before progressing to muscle weakness, difficult breathing, extreme hypotension, irregular heartbeat, and cardiac arrest. The risk of toxicity increases for those with impaired renal function and with kidney failure because the ability of the kidneys to remove magnesium is reduced or lost[136].

Excess Selenium

Selenium supplements and multivitamin/multimineral supplements that contain selenium in several forms are available. Researchers have proposed the use of brazil nuts, which contain very high amounts of selenium, as an alternative to selenium supplements and fortified foods. Six Brazil nuts, which weigh about 1 ounce, can contain 544 micrograms of selenium, or 780% of the Daily Value[137]. Brazil nuts can even be toxic if eaten regularly[138].

First indicators of excess selenium intake include garlic breath odor and metallic taste. Hair and nail loss or brittleness are signs of chronically high selenium intakes, aka selenosis. Other symptoms include lesions of the skin and nervous system, nausea, diarrhea, skin rashes, mottled teeth, fatigue, irritability, and nervous system abnormalities[139]. Acute selenium toxicity has resulted from ingestion of misformulated selenium products, including liquid supplements. Acute toxicity can cause severe gastrointestinal and neurological symptoms, acute respiratory distress syndrome, myocardial infarction, hair loss, muscle tenderness, tremors, lightheadedness, facial flushing, kidney failure, cardiac failure, and even death[140].

Excess Sodium

Humans began to use large amounts of salt for the main purpose of food preservation approximately 5,000 years ago and, although technologies have been developed since then allowing drastic reduction in the use of salt for food storage, excess dietary salt intake remains common.

Table salt, sodium chloride, is composed of about forty percent sodium and sixty percent chlorine. Sodium is the nutrient in salt and the primary element of concern. For decades there has been a lively, heated scientific debate over the dietary salt recommendations. The debate is among the most contentious in the field of nutrition. The health implications of excess salt intake is an area of continued investigations among scientists, clinicians, and public health experts[141].

Salt is pervasive in our food supply. According to the FDA, about twenty five percent of our salt intake comes from the natural salt in food and the salt we add while cooking and seasoning it. Over seventy five percent of the salt we eat is already in processed foods such as bread, breakfast cereal, and ready meals. Manufacturers continue to add salt to food products and cooks add salt to foods at restaurants and other food service establishments making excessive consumption hard to avoid for many people. Food product labels may have to be carefully examined to make the distinction between the salt and sodium contents. You can use the equations

Salt = 2.5 x sodium or

Sodium = 0.4 x salt

to figure out how much sodium you are eating.

Sea salt is produced from evaporation of water from oceans or lakes and with less processing than table salt. It comes in a variety of coarseness levels. Sea salt and table salt contain comparable amounts of sodium by weight and have the same basic nutritional value. The minerals in sea salt merely add flavor and color.

The ingestion of large amounts of salt may lead to nausea, vomiting, diarrhea, and abdominal cramps[142].

And it is worth remembering that dissolvable vitamin supplements and painkillers can contain a gram of salt per tablet. Many salt substitutes contain potassium chloride, which could be harmful to people with certain medical conditions such as diabetes, kidney disease, and heart disease.

In addition to excess table salt, be sure to avoid unnecessary and excess consumption of other commonly available sodium compounds such as monosodium glutamate (MSG), baking soda (sodium bicarbonate), baking powder (sodium bicarbonate plus one or more acid salts), and disodium phosphate.

Too much sodium in the diet can lead to high blood pressure, which is often called the silent killer because it typically has no symptoms until after it has done significant damage to the heart and arteries. It has been estimated that one out of five Americans and one out of three people in England have high blood pressure and don't even know they are at risk for heart attack, stroke, heart failure, kidney disease, and eye disease. If you haven't already done so, you should get your blood pressure tested.

Dietary salt appears to be an important single factor in raising the blood pressure[143]. A recent study actually observed and confirmed that the risk of developing hypertension is greater in people with relatively high dietary sodium consumption compared with those with relatively low sodium intake. The study demonstrated that both a relatively high level of dietary sodium intake and a gradual increase in dietary sodium are associated with a future increase in blood pressure and incidence of hypertension in the general population.

Processed Meat and Sodium

Human nutritional epidemiology is considered an important tool in making dietary recommendations. A study that is often cited appeared online May 17, 2010, on the website of the journal Circulation. Researchers at the Harvard School of Public Health systematically reviewed nearly 1,600 studies. Twenty relevant studies were identified, which included a total of 1,218,380 individuals from 10 countries on four continents (North America, Europe, Australia, and Asia). The results showed that, on average, each daily serving of processed meat (about 1-2 slices of deli meats or 1 hot dog) was associated with a 42% higher risk of developing heart disease and a 19% higher risk of developing diabetes. In contrast, eating unprocessed red meat was not associated with risk of developing heart disease or diabetes.

When they looked at average nutrients in unprocessed red and processed meats eaten in the United States, researchers found that they contained similar average amounts of saturated fat and cholesterol. In contrast, processed meats contained, on average, 400% more sodium and 50% more nitrate preservatives. This suggested that differences in salt and preservatives, rather than fats, might explain the higher risk of heart disease and diabetes seen with processed meats, but not with unprocessed red meats.

Acknowledging that cause-and-effect cannot be proven by these types of long-term observational studies, the authors concluded that the predicted blood-pressure effects of the high sodium content alone can account for more than 2/3 of the observed relationship between processed meats and cardiovascular disease risk[144].

A later study published in BMC Medicine involving 448,568 participants in 10 European countries, showed that intake of unprocessed red meat was not significantly associated with total or cause-specific mortality; conversely, intake of processed meat was associated with a 30% higher rate of cardiovascular disease and also higher cancer mortality. The findings were consistent with previous meta-analysis, based on smaller studies, showing strong associations of processed meats, but not unprocessed meats, with cardiovascular disease. The authors concluded that dietary recommendations should continue to move away from fat-based guidelines and instead focus upon foods and dietary patterns, including increased consumption of fruits, vegetables, nuts, whole grains, and fish, and avoidance of processed meats, other high-sodium foods, partially hydrogenated vegetable oils, and refined grains, starches, and sugars[145].

The authors also concluded *"The fact that a mild increase in sodium intake within the range observed in usual daily life but not a drastic sodium load, as observed in interventional studies, increases the chance of developing hypertension may become a driving force for the reduction of dietary sodium consumption in the general population. Furthermore, an effort not to increase dietary sodium as well as an effort to reduce dietary sodium intake may be effective for the primary prevention of hypertension or reduction of blood pressure in the population at large."*[146]

Through its effects on hypertension, salt is a major risk factor for stroke mortality[147]. Worldwide, hypertension is the leading preventable risk factor for death and causes 54% of strokes.

In renal disease, a high salt intake accelerates the rate of renal functional deterioration.

Many epidemiological studies have analyzed the relationship between excess salt intake and risk of gastric cancer. Altogether, epidemiological, clinical, and experimental evidence supports the possibility of a substantial reduction in the rates of gastric cancer through progressive reduction in population salt intake[148].

Excess Zinc

Excessive zinc can suppress rather than stimulate the immune system.

Dietary zinc supplements contain several forms of zinc, and the percentage of elemental zinc varies with the form. The elemental zinc content should be provided on the Supplemental Facts panel of a product's container.

Acute zinc toxicity can result in nausea, vomiting, loss of appetite, abdominal cramps, diarrhea, and headaches. The major consequence of long-term consumption of excessive zinc is copper deficiency.

Other chronic effects include altered iron function, and reduced immune function. Excessive zinc supplementation suppresses immune function by interfering with copper absorption, leading to copper deficiency, anemia, changes in red and white blood cells and lowered immunity. Chronically high intakes might possibly affect some aspects of urinary physiology[149].

Making Informed Decisions on Dietary Supplements

By law, any product labeled as a dietary supplement must carry a Supplement Facts panel that list its contents and other added ingredients (such as fillers, binders, and flavorings). In June 2013, the government launched the Dietary Supplement Label Database (DSLD). Hosted by the National Institutes of Health, the database is available at the DSLD website. The link is provided at endnote number 150 in the References[150]. The DSLD contains information taken from the labels of tens of thousands dietary supplement products available in the U.S. marketplace. The DSLD offers these features:

- **Quick Search:** Search for any ingredient or specific text on a label.
- **Search for Dietary Ingredients:** An alphabetical list of ingredients is provided.
- **Search for Specific Products:** An alphabetical list of products is provided.
- **Browse Contact Information:** Search by supplement manufacturer or distributor.
- **Advanced Search:** Search by using a combination of search options including dietary ingredient, product/brand name, health-related claims, and label statements.

The DSLD is updated regularly to incorporate new dietary supplements that are added to the marketplace each year, products that are removed, and product formulations that are adjusted, as is the information on their labels.

Consumers are cautioned by the FDA that dietary supplements, in general, are not FDA-approved. Under the law (Dietary Supplement Health and Education Act of 1994), dietary supplement firms do not need FDA approval prior to marketing their products. It is the company's responsibility to make sure its products are safe and that any claims are true.

FDA warns the just because you see a supplement product on a store shelf does not mean it is safe or effective. When safety issues are suspected, FDA must investigate and, when warranted, take steps to have the product removed from the market. However, it is much easier for a firm to get a product on the market than it is for FDA to take a product off the market.

Finally, if you are taking supplements, make sure you are aware of the tolerable upper limit of the vitamins and minerals you're taking, and check all labels to make sure your food choices are not enriched with the same nutrients. **Your best option is to avoid supplements unless your doctor advises you to take them and be sure you understand the reasons for his/her recommendation.**

Food Additives

A food additive is any substance added to food. The FDA's database titled, "Everything Added to Food in the United States," contains over 3,000 ingredients. Legally the term refers to *"any substance the intended use of which results or may reasonably be expected to result – directly or indirectly – in its becoming a component or otherwise affecting the characteristics of any food."* The purpose of that definition is to impose a premarket approval requirement. The definition excludes ingredients that don't require government approval because they are generally recognized to be safe, and ingredients approved by use by the FDA or USDA prior to the 1958 law, and color additives and pesticides where other legal premarket approval requirements apply. Food manufacturers are required to list all ingredients in the food on the label. However, some ingredients don't have to be listed individually and can be listed collectively as *"flavors," "spices," "artificial flavoring,"* or *"artificial colors,"* for color additives exempt from certification.

The eighteen classes of additives include (preservatives), (sweeteners), (color additives), (flavors and spices), (flavor enhancers), (fat replacers), (nutrients), (emulsifiers), (stabilizers and thickeners, binders, texturizers), (pH control agents and acidulates), (leavening agents), (anti-caking agents), (humectants), (yeast nutrients), (dough strengtheners and conditioners), (firming agents), (enzyme preparations), and gases (carbon dioxide and nitrous oxide).

The reader is encouraged to visit the FDA website at the link provided in endnote number 151 in the References[151] for information concerning the purpose of the additives (what they are supposed to do), example of their uses, and names found on product labels. For instance, under the category of (stabilizers and thickeners, binders, texturizers), the purposes of the additives are: to produce uniform texture, improve *"mouth-feel."* Examples of their use include frozen desserts, dairy products, cakes, pudding and gelatin mixes, dressings, jams and jellies, and sauces. The names found on product labels are gelatin, pectin, guar gum, carrageenan, xanthan gum, and whey.

As you might expect there is a great deal of controversy regarding the regulations and the safety of food additives. Of particular concern to NRDC (a nonprofit organization devoted to protecting health and the environment) and many others is the gaping loophole *"…ingredients that don't require government approval because they are generally recognized to be safe,"* that goes by the abbreviation **GRAS**. According to the NRDC:

" The exemption allows manufacturers to make safety determinations that the uses of their newest chemicals in food are safe without notifying the FDA. The agency's attempts to limit these undisclosed GRAS determinations by asking industry to voluntarily inform the FDA about their chemicals are insufficient to ensure the safety of our food in today's global marketplace with a complex food supply."[152]

Many of the FDA approved additives are controversial. The thousand of additives are too numerous to list and discuss in this book. Among the most controversial are artificial sweeteners, artificial colors, BHA, sodium nitrite, and sodium benzoate.

Artificial Sweeteners

According to the Nutrition Source at the Harvard School of Public Health, *"There is conflicting research surrounding the health benefits of artificially sweetened drinks. Long-term studies show that regular consumption of artificially sweetened beverages reduces the intake of calories and promotes weight loss or maintenance, but other research shows no effect, and some studies even show weight gain."*[153]

Most diet or low-calorie food products are made using artificial sweeteners including aspartame, sucralose, saccharine, Stevia, acesulfame K, neotame, and cyclamates. The artificial sweeteners aspartame, acesulfame K, saccharine, neotame, and sucralose are all FDA approved. Cyclamates are banned in the United States because they were shown to cause bladder cancer in animals.

During premarket review, FDA established an acceptable daily intake (ADI) level for each of the five high-intensity sweeteners approved as food additives. An ADI is the amount of a substance that is considered safe to consume each day over the course of a person's lifetime. For each of these sweeteners, FDA determined that the estimated daily intake even for a high consumer of the substance would not exceed the ADI. Generally, an additive does not present safety concerns if the estimated daily intake is less than the ADI. The ADIs can be found in the Summary Table published by the FDA on their website. The link for their website can be found at endnote number 154 in the References[154].

FDA has not permitted the use of whole-leaf Stevia or crude Stevia extracts because these substances have not been approved for use as a food additive. FDA does not consider their use in food to be GRAS in light of reports in the literature that raise concerns about the use of these substances. Among these concerns are control of blood sugar and effects on the reproductive, cardiovascular, and renal systems. The food additives and GRAS affirmation petition or pre-petition submissions for the use of such substances that FDA has received in the past have not contained the data and information necessary to establish the safe use of these substances as ingredients in food[155].

The FDA only approves or denies approval to foods and food additives, not **supplements**. The agency has declined to grant stevia approval as a food additive, but it does not regulate stevia as a dietary supplement. Because of this, health food stores and natural food stores can sell whole stevia and crude extracts of stevia without needing FDA approval as long as they label it as a dietary supplement, not as a food.

The FDA has made an exception for products derived from a specific component of stevia. The compound Rebaudioside A differs from Stevia in that it is a highly purified product. Products marketed as *"Stevia"* are whole leaf Stevia or Stevia extracts of which Rebaudioside A is a component[156].

According to Stevia.net: *"The U.S. Food and Drug Administration since the mid-1980s has labeled stevia an "unsafe food additive" and gone to extensive lengths to keep it off the U.S. market — including initiating a search-and-seizure campaign and full-fledged "import alert"... So adamant has the FDA remained on the subject, that even though stevia can now be legally marketed as a dietary supplement under legislation enacted in 1994, any mention of its possible use as a sweetener or tea is still strictly prohibited."* [157]

There are other sugar substitutes in addition to the high-intensity sweeteners. Sugar alcohols, another class of sweeteners, can be used as sugar substitutes. Examples include sorbitol, xylitol, lactitol, mannitol, erythritol, and maltitol. The sweetness of sugar alcohols varies from 25% to 100% as sweet as sugar. Sugar alcohols are slightly lower in calories than sugar and do not promote tooth decay or cause a sudden increase in blood glucose. They are used primarily to sweeten sugar-free candies, cookies, and chewing gums.

Color Additives or Food Dyes

Candy, soft drinks, breakfast cereals, frozen desserts and even salad dressings all contain artificial coloring agents. They are used to make products attractive, appealing, and appetizing. Color additives are not supposed to be used deceptively as in masking a spoiled, damaged, or inferior product.

By definition, a color additive is any dye, pigment or substance which when added or applied to a food is capable – alone or through reactions with other substances – of imparting color. FDA is responsible for regulating all color additives to ensure that foods containing color additives are safe to eat, contain only approved ingredients, and are accurately labeled.

Color additives are either certified or exempt from certification. Both types are subjected to safety and toxicology tests. *"Certifiable"* color additives are man-made. Those classified as certifiable must be submitted by the manufacturer for batch certification by FDA. If FDA *"certifies"* the batch it issues a certification lot number. Only then can that batch be used legally in FDA-regulated products. When a new batch is deemed acceptable for use in foods, its common name is changed according to the following naming convention: the acronym FD&C, a color, and a number, e.g., FD&C Red No. 40, or FD&C Yellow No. 6, which is often found in cereals, ice cream, and baked goods. Sometimes a color additive is identified by a shortened form of its name, consisting of just the color and number, such as Yellow 6.

Currently, there are nine colorings on the list, seven of which are approved for use in foods in the United States. They are: FD&C Blue No. 1, FD&C Blue No. 2, FD&C Green No. 3, FD&C Red No. 40, FD&C Red No. 3, FD&C Yellow No. 5, and FD&C Yellow No. 6.

The other two are used to color casings or surfaces of frankfurters and sausages (Orange B) and the skins of oranges not used for processing (Citrus Red No. 2).

In recent years, others such as FD&C Red No. 2, FD&C Red No. 4, and FD&C Red No. 32, to name a few were banned for use due to adverse health effects. Color additives that FDA has found to cause cancer in animals or humans may not be used in FDA-regulated products marketed in the United States.

Color additives exempt from certification, meaning that they do not undergo batch certification, are largely derived from plant, animal, or mineral sources. These include annatto extract, caramel, beta-carotene, grape skin extract, turmeric, paprika oleoresin, and others. Some of the exempt color additives, like beta-carotene, are also made synthetically, and those in the industry often refer to these as *nature-identical colorings*. They are not subject to batch certification requirements, but they are still artificial color additives and must comply with regulatory requirements. The rationale is that if a color additive, regardless of its derivation, is not inherent to the food product, that product has been colored artificially.

Food ingredients such as cherries, green or red peppers, chocolate, and orange juice, which contribute their own natural color when mixed with other foods, are not regarded as color additives, but where a food substance such as beet juice is deliberately used as a color, as in pink lemonade, it is a color additive.

Certified color additives are listed on ingredient declarations by their certified name, e.g. FD&C Red No. 40, but it is not necessary to include *"FD&C"* or *"No."* on the declaration. Exempt color additives may be listed as *"artificial color," "artificial color added,"* or *"color added"* or a term that indicates a coloring was used, as well as "colored with *"X"* or *"X color,"* with X being the name of the color additive.

There is no *"generally recognized as safe"* (GRAS) exemption to the definition of a color additive. However, a substance that is listed as GRAS also may be listed as a color additive, but the use of the substance as a color additive (in addition to its use as a GRAS substance) would require premarket approval by FDA[158].

The topic of food additives and their possible health effects is highly controversial. One noted controversy that has persisted for more than 40 years is that synthetic color additives can adversely affect behavior in children, particularly those diagnosed with Attention Deficit Disorder (ADD) and Attention Deficit Hyperactivity Disorder (ADHD). Additionally, critics cite studies that link food dyes to allergies and cancer.[159]

The Mayo Clinic states that there's no solid evidence that food additives cause ADHD, but admits it is a controversial topic. While some studies indicate that certain food colorings and preservatives may increase hyperactive behavior in some children, the FDA Food Advisory Committee determined that studies to date have not proved there's a link between food colorings and hyperactivity[160].

FDA critics point out that *"in the United States, children can drink fruit juice beverages made with Red Dye No. 40 and eat macaroni and cheese colored with Yellow Dye No. 5 and No. 6. Yet in the U.K., these artificial colorings have been taken off the market due to health concerns, and in the rest of Europe, products that contain them must carry labels warning of the dyes' potential adverse effect on children's attention and behavior."* [161]

To critics the differences in U.S. and European regulations underscores the differences in the policy approaches of the governments in the U.S. and Europe.

The European Union's chemicals management and environmental protection policies are based on the precautionary principle. This principle, in the words of the European Commission, *"aims at ensuring a higher level of environmental protection through "preventative"* decision-making. In other words, when there is substantial, credible evidence of danger to human or environmental health, protective action should be taken despite continuing scientific uncertainty.

In contrast, the U.S. federal government's approach to chemicals management sets a high bar for the proof of harm that must be demonstrated before regulatory action is taken. And, critics argue, current U.S. policies require cost-benefit analyses with high bars for proof of harm rather than a proof of safety for entry onto the market.

European and U.S. authorities reached different conclusions in the case of Red Dye No. 40, Yellow Dye No. 5 and Yellow Dye No. 6 after considering the same evidence reported in a 2007 double-blind study by U.K. researchers that found that eating artificially colored food appeared to increase children's hyperactivity. In the U.K., the authorities barred use of these dyes as food additives. The EU chose to require warning labels on products that contain them. In the U.S., the FDA found the study inconclusive because it looked at effects of a mixture of additives rather than individual colorings.

In countries where these food colors and dyes are banned, food companies employ natural colorants instead, such as paprika extract, beetroot, and annatto[162].

Preservatives BHA and BHT

BHA (butylated hydroxyanisole) and BHT (butylated hydroxytoluene) are antioxidants used to slow the spoilage of certain fats and oils in food. The common preservatives protect the flavor, color and odor of processed foods such as butters, meats, crackers, nut mixes, cereals, chewing gum, baked goods, vitamins, dehydrated potatoes, potato chips, and beer, and they prevent the oxidation of some nutrients. BHA and BHT may also have antiviral and antimicrobial properties. BHT has been mentioned anecdotally as beneficial in the treatment of herpes simplex and possibly AIDS[163]. BHT is sold in supplements as an antioxidant.

There's ongoing controversy about the safety of BHA and BHT as a food preservative. The Food and Drug Administration (FDA) categorizes these food additives as GRAS—Generally Recognized As Safe—which means they are widely considered safe for their intended use in specified amounts, but do not have to undergo pre-market review. A review by an independent committee supported their general safety, but concluded that *"uncertainties exist, requiring that additional studies be conducted."* Most research has been conducted with animals and in test tubes, not in people.

Based on animal studies, the National Toxicology Program has concluded that BHA *"is reasonably anticipated to be a human carcinogen,"* while BHT has been linked to an increased—or sometimes decreased—risk of cancer in animals.

The National Institutes of Health said that although studies show BHA can induce cancer in rats, existing scientific literature is *"inadequate to evaluate the relationship between human cancer and the exposure specifically to BHA."*

BHA and BHT have biological effects, some which may be harmful, and some which may be beneficial. Some lab and animal studies have found that BHA and BHT—at high levels as well as at lower levels found in foods—may have anti-cancer properties, possibly through the scavenging of damaging free radicals or by stimulating production of enzymes that detoxify carcinogens. Other research suggests that low doses of BHA are toxic to cells, while high doses are protective—or the reverse, that low doses are okay, but high doses are harmful. In other words, no one really knows how BHA and BHT react in the human body.

The FDA concluded that a 2000 study found consumption of BHA and BHT does not increase people's risk of stomach cancer and may actually reduce it.

BHA Cancer Studies in Humans

The data available from epidemiological studies are inadequate to evaluate the relationship between human cancer and exposure specifically to BHA. Since BHA was listed in the Sixth Annual Report on Carcinogens, one epidemiological study of BHA has been identified. A population-based nested case-control study of stomach cancer in men and women within the Netherlands Cohort Study of dietary intake found no increase in risk at typical levels of dietary intake of BHA (Botterweck et al. 2000).[164]

FDA's position is that *"BHA is generally recognized as safe for use in food when the total of antioxidants is not greater than 0.02% of fat or oil content. BHA may be used as a food additive permitted for direct addition to food for human consumption as prescribed in 21 CFR 172 and 166. BHA may be used in the manufacture of food packaging materials, with a limit of addition to food of 0.005%. BHA may be used as an antioxidant in defoaming agents for processed foods, not to exceed 0.1% by weight of defoamer."*

Consumers who are concerned about the safety of BHA or BHT may wish to choose products that use other preservatives such as Vitamin E or rosemary oil.

Rosemary oil, an alternative antioxidant, has been touted as a natural foods replacement for synthetic antioxidants in foods. The antioxidant activity of the plant is attributed to their phenolic compound content, which includes volatile compounds also known as essential oils. Rosemary oil is listed by the FDA for Generally Recognized as Safe (GRAS) food use.

Given the uncertainty regarding the safety of BHA and BHT, you may choose to avoid products with preservatives and eat fresh and minimally processed foods, which contain few or no additives.[165]

Nitrites and Nitrates

Approximately 80% of dietary nitrates are derived from the consumption of leafy vegetables. Nitrites are produced internally from nitric oxide (NO) and through the conversion of nitrates (NO_3^-) to nitrites (NO_2^-) by bacteria in the mouth and gastrointestinal tract. Drinking water also contributes very small amounts of nitrate and nitrite. Nitrates have one nitrogen atom and three oxygen atoms, while nitrites have two oxygen atoms[166].

Sodium Nitrite

Sodium nitrite ($NaNO_2^-$) is a food additive and preservative commonly used in cured meats. It is used in refrigerated meats to inhibit the growth of microorganisms that can cause the fatal food poisoning botulism. It also can extend the storage life of meat by inhibiting the growth of some other disease causing microorganisms such as Listeria. Nitrite is also used to change the color of meat to desirable shades of red. For example, the pinkish color in cured and emulsion meats like ham, sausages, and hot dogs. And it also imparts a unique taste to cured meats. Sodium nitrite acts as an antioxidant to delay the development of oxidative rancidity.

Sodium Nitrite is toxic in high amounts. Charring or overcooking meats containing sodium nitrite can create carcinogenic nitrosamines. Carcinogenic nitrosamines can also be formed during the curing process.

The FDA regulates allowable levels of inorganic nitrite in foodstuffs as well as in bottled water. The bottled water standard is based on the EPA standards for tap water.

The FDA prescribes conditions that regulate the safe use of sodium nitrite as a color fixative in smoked cured tuna fish products; as a preservative and color fixative, with or without sodium nitrate, in smoked, cured sablefish, smoked, cured salmon, and smoked, cured shad; and as a preservative and color fixative, with sodium nitrate, in meat-curing preparations for the home curing of meat and meat products (including poultry and wild game). The agency also regulates its use in canned pet food containing meat and fish.[167]

The USDA also regulates nitrates and nitrites. The USDA classifies nitrates and nitrites as curing agents because of their biological reactivity, and it classifies them as preservatives because nitrates and nitrites retard bacteria growth that spoils food and causes illness.

The USDA regulations define when nitrate/nitrite is required, allowed, or prohibited. The regulations prohibit the use of purified nitrate and nitrite in _Organic_ meat products. _Natural_ meat products also are not allowed to use nitrate and nitrite.

The USDA permits the manufacture of uncured versions of typically cured meats. _Uncured_ meat products do not contain nitrate or nitrite, even though traditionally required or expected to contain curing ingredients (e.g. products like frankfurters and bologna). _Traditional_ meat products may be required to contain curing ingredients – nitrate and/or nitrite – but some products (e.g. turkey breast) are not required to do so although the manufacturer may choose add them.

Vegetables high in naturally accumulating nitrate and nitrite (such as celery) are now commonly used to cure meat products with a natural, plant based source for curing. However, products cured using plant-based nitrate and nitrite are required to be labeled *"uncured."* That's because the amount of nitrite that forms from nitrate in the celery powder or juice is difficult to monitor; the nitrites found in products cured with the celery powder or juice could contain less nitrites or vastly greater amounts than found in products cured with the purified sodium nitrite. This makes the risk for nitrosamine formation or bacterial contamination in the plant based version more challenging to evaluate. And it can create confusion so you have to read the labels carefully.

If cured with a purified source, you will see the words *"sodium nitrite"* on the label. If cured with a natural source, you will see the words *"celery powder"* or other similar vegetable ingredients on the label instead[168].

If you want to reduce the nitrosamines in your diet, avoid or limit your consumption of processed meats.

Sodium Nitrate

Sodium nitrate ($NaNO_3^-$) is a food additive used as a preservative and color fixative in cured meats and smoked foods, like sausage, hotdogs, ham, and poultry. It has also been used to preserve fish and vegetables. Nitrate serves as a _precursor_ to nitrite. Nitrate is only effective as a curing ingredient if first reduced to nitrite. Dietary nitrate from vegetable consumption, for example, has been shown to serve as a significant source for the internal production of nitrite and nitric oxide in the human body. Nitrate _per se_ is relatively non-toxic, but its metabolites and reaction products e.g. nitrite, nitric oxide, and N-nitroso compounds, have raised concern because of implications for adverse health effects such as methemoglobinemia and carcinogenesis[169].

The external sources for human intake of nitrate are primarily derived from plant derived foods and drinking water with approximately 80% of total nitrate intake being attributed to food and another 14% to water. Vegetables actually constitute a large component of the dietary intake of nitrate. The National Academy of Sciences[170] reported that 87% of dietary nitrate intake associated with food is derived from vegetables. Overall, the estimated exposures to nitrate from vegetables are unlikely to result in appreciable health risks.

Many food components are beneficial at low and harmful at high intakes. Researchers have shown that the consumption of nitrate- and nitrite-containing plant foods have beneficial health effects and have questioned the rationale of proposals to limit nitrate and nitrite consumption from plant foods.[171]

The FDA prescribes conditions that regulate the safe use of sodium nitrate as preservative and color fixative, with or without sodium nitrite, in smoked cured sablefish, smoked, cured salmon, and smoked, cured shad; as a preservative and color fixative, with or without sodium nitrite, in meat-curing preparations for the home curing of meat and meat products (including poultry and wild game)[172].

Although nitrates and nitrites have been used for curing meat for many centuries, acute toxic effects have only been encountered at very high doses. The toxicity reported has been principally methemoglobinemia, but only when several grams of nitrate salt are administered. Some early studies may have shown methemoglobinemia with lower doses of nitrate due to contamination with nitrite. Nitrite causes acute toxicity in much smaller doses.

It is possible that certain subgroups of the human population may be at increased risk of cancer if subject to high levels of dietary nitrate.

Methemoglobinemia

The major acute toxic effect of nitrate and nitrite poisoning is methemoglobinemia, a blood disorder in which an abnormal amount of methemoglobin – a form of hemoglobin – is produced. A most common cause of methemoglobinemia is the ingestion or inhalation of nitrates or nitrites. Well water contaminated by nitrogenous fertilizer run-off is an important cause of nitrate-induced methemoglobinemia.

Methemoglobin reduces the oxygen-carrying capacity of the blood and in addition, it increases the affinity of the remaining hemoglobin to oxygen. The remaining hemoglobin is able to bind oxygen molecules more efficiently, but it is less able to release oxygen to tissues.

Nausea, vomiting and abdominal pain may occur. Tachycardia, hypotension and collapse may also occur. Stupor, coma and convulsions have been seen to occur in severe poisoning due to severe hypoxia[173].

Exposure to nitrates and nitrites at levels above health-based risk values has been reported to have adverse health effects on infants and children. Note, however, that the few human nitrate and nitrite exposure studies including children and adults have not produced methemoglobinemia. The greatest risk of nitrate poisoning occurs in infants fed well water contaminated with nitrates[174].

Nitrites in the body promote blood clotting, regulate blood pressure and boost immune function. Nitrate and nitrite play a role in modulating blood pressure in both health and disease states.

A study was published in the New England Journal of Medicine in December 2006 by researchers in Sweden that examined the effects of dietary nitrate on blood pressure in healthy volunteers. The researchers conclude that short-term dietary supplementation with inorganic nitrate reduces diastolic blood pressure in healthy young volunteers.[175]

A later study (2012) by an Australian research group used beetroot juice as a source of inorganic nitrate. They found that the consumption of beetroot juice on a low nitrate diet may lower blood pressure and therefore reduce the risk of cardiovascular events. However, it is unknown if its inclusion as part of a normal diet has a similar effect on blood pressure[176].

Sodium Benzoate

Sodium benzoate, the sodium salt of benzoic acid, is widely used as a preservative in pharmaceutical preparations, foods (e.g. pickles, salsa and dip) and soft drinks. Under acidic conditions, sodium benzoate inhibits growth of bacteria, mold and yeast, extending a product's shelf life.

Benzoic acid occurs naturally in many plants and in animals. It is therefore a natural constituent of many foods, including milk products. While benzoic acid is found naturally in low levels in cranberries, prunes, plums, cinnamon, ripe cloves, most berries, and other foods, the sodium benzoate listed on a product's nutrition label is typically synthesized by the reaction of benzoic acid with sodium hydroxide, which makes it dissolve in water.

After oral uptake, sodium benzoate is rapidly absorbed from the gastrointestinal tract and metabolized in the liver resulting in the formation of hippuric acid. Hippurate is rapidly excreted in the urine. Owing to rapid metabolism and excretion, the accumulation of the benzoates or their metabolites is not expected to occur[177].

The ingestion of sodium benzoate at the Generally Regarded as Safe (GRAS) dose is known to lead to a robust excursion in the plasma hippurate level. Some past research demonstrated adverse effects of benzoate and hippurate on glucose homeostasis in cells and in animal models, leading researchers to hypothesize that benzoate might represent a widespread and underappreciated diabetogenic dietary exposure in humans. When they evaluated whether acute exposure to GRAS levels of sodium benzoate alters insulin and glucose homeostasis through a randomized, controlled, cross-over study of 14 overweight subjects, they did not find a statistically significant effect of an acute oral exposure to sodium benzoate on glucose homeostasis. Although their study showed that GRAS doses of benzoate do not have an acute, adverse effect on glucose homeostasis, they concluded that future studies will be necessary to explore the metabolic impact of chronic benzoate exposure[178].

The Food and Drug Administration limits sodium benzoate to concentrations of 0.1% by weight, but most foods have concentrations far lower –more like 0.025% to 0.05%. Therefore, some university scientists have stated that sodium benzoate poses no great health dangers, when consumed under normal conditions[179].

In humans, the acute toxicity of sodium benzoate is low. However, when sodium benzoate combines with ascorbic acid (vitamin C) benzene can form, which is a known carcinogen. The rate at which benzene is formed is affected by light and heat, as well as the time spent on a shelf from production to consumption.

It has been known for a long time that benzene can form at very low levels (parts per billion) in some beverages that contain both benzoate salts and ascorbic acid (vitamin C) or erythorbic acid (a closely related substance (isomer) also known as d-ascorbic acid). The vitamin C can be present naturally in beverages or added to prevent spoilage or to provide additional nutrients.

The FDA first became aware that benzene was present in some soft drinks in 1990. At that time, the soft drink industry informed the agency that benzene could form at low levels in some beverages that contained both benzoate salts and ascorbic acid. Subsequently, the FDA and the beverage industry initiated research to identify factors contributing to benzene formation. As a result, many manufacturers reformulated their products to reduce or eliminate benzene formation.

But in November 2005, FDA received reports that benzene had been detected at low levels in some soft drinks containing benzoate salts and ascorbic acid. As a result the FDA Center for Food Safety and Applied Nutrition, initiated a survey of benzene levels in soft drinks and other beverages. The vast majority of the beverages sampled to date (including those containing both benzoate salts and ascorbic acid) contained either no detectable benzene or levels well below the 5 ppb EPA maximum contaminant level for benzene in drinking water[180].

Spices

Spices have been important to mankind since the beginning of history. *"Pen Ts'ao Ching"* or *"The Classic Herbal"* written around 2700 BC mentioned more than a hundred medicinal plants including the spice cassia, which is similar to cinnamon. Today, spices are primarily used for and associated with adding to or enhancing the flavor of foods including meats, sauces, vegetables and desserts. Most spices are derived from bark (e.g. cinnamon), fruit (e.g. red and black pepper), and seed (e.g. nutmeg) of plants.

The FDA defines spices as aromatic vegetable substances, in the whole, broken, or ground form, whose significant function in food is seasoning rather than nutrition.

The FDA first issued advisory standards in 1918 that defined the collective term "spices" and described a number of specific foods classified as spices. The advisory standards provided substantial guidance to the food industry concerning acceptable labeling of spices or flavorings, and foods in which these were used. And they were useful as guides to regulatory officials.

The advisory standards were later considered in connection with preparation of the list of *"Generally Recognized As Safe"* (GRAS) spices and other natural flavorings, and in the promulgation of regulations concerning food labeling.

The FDA also issued descriptions for 38 commonly used spices to provide guidance concerning acceptable names for use in labeling spices and foods in which they are used. Only the commonly used spices are included. For example, in the case of cinnamon, which will be discussed below, the FDA description is:

CINNAMON (Cassia) - The dried bark of Cinnamomum zeylanicum Sees (Ceylon cinnamon), Cinnamomum cassia Blume (Chinese cinnamon), or Cinnamomum loureirii Nees (Saigon cinnamon). It is brown to reddish-brown in color. The principal active ingredient in the volatile oil is cinnamaldehyde, which is responsible for the characteristic odor...

The description for the other 37 spices can be found on the FDA website at the link furnished in endnote number 181 in the References[181].

The FDA does not consider poppy seeds, sesame seeds, dried or dehydrated onions and garlic to be spices. (Onions, garlic, shallots, leeks, and chives are alliums) The spices paprika, turmeric and saffron are *"color"* as well as spices. When used as ingredients in foods they must be designated as *"spice and coloring,"* unless each is designated by its specific name.

Some plants that are processed into foods often contain natural substances that may be hazardous to human health. One example is coumarin, which is known to cause liver and kidney damage in rats, mice and probably humans. Coumarin is not a spice. It is a chemical found in tonka beans and widespread in plants including many vegetables, fruits, and medicinal plants. Coumarin has a vanilla-like aroma and taste and it is an anticoagulant.

The FDA, and many sister agencies around the globe, banned coumarin as a food additive decades ago. Coumarin was banned as a food additive in the United States in 1954. It is currently listed by FDA among *"Substances Generally Prohibited From Direct Addition or Use as Human Food.* Though its damage is not permanent, it is generally recognized that it is important to limit coumarin consumption. Coumarin is used to produce low priced imitation *"vanilla extract."* Real vanilla doesn't contain coumarin. The infamous *"bargain"* Mexican vanilla in addition to being sold in Mexico and other Latin American countries was a coumarin-containing product that once appeared on the shelves of some U.S. stores. Concerns regarding the health effects of coumarin prompted the FDA to issue an alert in 2008 about the fraudulent vanilla extract being sold to tourists in Mexico[182].

> **Coumarin**
>
> The name Coumarin comes from the Tupi word for the name of the Tonka bean tree, a species of flowering tree in the pea family. Tonka beans were once considered to be the major source of coumarin.
>
> Coumarins are widespread in plants including many vegetables, spices, fruits, and medicinal plants. Most of these compounds are not harmful to humans in the amounts present in edible plants. Coumarin had been used as a flavoring agent in food, alcoholic beverages and tobacco.
>
> Evidence of the hepatotoxic effects of this compound in animal models led the FDA to ban coumarin as a food flavoring agent. Human clinical data indicated that a majority of people were less sensitive to coumarin than the rodent models used to investigate the toxic effects of this compound. However, a particular group of the population was found to be more susceptible to coumarin-induced hepatotoxicity.
>
> Ingesting substantial amounts of coumarin on a daily basis may pose a health risk to individuals who are more sensitive to this compound.

Trace quantities of coumarin are found in cinnamon bark of Cinnamomum zeylanicum (zeylanicum is the Latin word for Ceylon) but the cassia bark *Cinnamomum cassia* contains a much higher concentration. The levels of coumarin in cassia cinnamon vary greatly even in bark from the same tree. One study showed that, on average, cassia cinnamon powder had 63 times more coumarin than Ceylon cinnamon powder[183].

Various comparisons exist for estimated concentrations. One of them estimates Ceylon cinnamon has between 2-5 parts per million of coumarin compared to 2000-5000 parts per million for cassia. Another estimates one teaspoon of cassia cinnamon powder contains 5.8 to 12.1 mg of coumarin, which is close to the Tolerable Daily Intake level in Germany.

Even though coumarin as such or as a constituent of tonka beans or tonka extracts is listed under the substances generally prohibited from direct addition or use as human food in the U.S., coumarin content in cassia cinnamon-flavored food is not regulated as in Europe. Most of the cinnamon sold in the U.S. is cassia cinnamon, with prices one third to one tenth of Ceylon cinnamon.

Germany's Federal Institute for Risk Assessment (BfR) has warned that anyone who regularly eats a lot of cassia cinnamon—more than two grams (0.07 ounce) a day for a 132-pound adult—could be at risk for side effects. BfR doesn't have any reports of side effects from occasional consumption of cinnamon. The BfR recommends Cassia cinnamon for moderate consumption and Ceylon cinnamon for consumers who frequently use large quantities of cinnamon as a condiment.

In the past, the medicinal uses of spices (and herbs) were often indistinguishable from their culinary uses; people have recognized for centuries both the potential toxicity, as well as inherent value, of phytochemicals in relation to human health[184].

And there is a growing body of literature concerning the potential/purported benefits of these foods from a health perspective. These benefits include their possible role in conferring protection against neurodegenerative diseases, cardiovascular disease, cancer, and type 2 diabetes.

On the other hand, there are also data suggesting that some spices may increase cancer risk. Several case-control studies in India have observed that gastrointestinal cancer risk was higher with consumption of spicy foods and chili[185].

From a culinary perspective spices (and herbs) can be used in recipes to partially or wholly replace less desirable ingredients such as salt, sugar and added saturated fat in, for example, marinades and dressings, stir-fry dishes, casseroles, soups, curries and Mediterranean-style cooking. Vegetable dishes and vegetarian options may be more appetizing when prepared with spices (and herbs)[186].

Variety and Moderation

Moderate consumption is a good practice for any substances that you eat, particularly those that you consume on a frequent basis. Eating the same foods on a daily basis can permit the accumulation of toxins that are present in trace amounts. This especially applies to plant based substances. It is a good practice to vary your diet so you don't eat the same food items every day. For example, experts warn that consumption of Brazil nuts on a daily basis should be limited to no more than a few nuts to avoid accumulation of selenium in the tissues[187]. And high potassium foods such as fennel should be consumed in moderation when taking beta-blockers, which can cause potassium levels to increase in the blood. High levels of potassium in the body can pose a serious risk to those with kidney damage or kidneys that are not fully functional. Damaged kidneys may be unable to filter excess potassium from the blood, which could be fatal[188].

The closing advice in this chapter is to stress the importance to review reliable information about their safety and interactions before you use additives and supplements. When possible, choose fresh foods rather than those that have been processed with additives for a longer shelf life or to fulfill other requirements of modern food production.

Continue to avoid foods that you may like but make you ill, like spicy foods or fatty foods that cause diarrhea, and don't eat foods for which you have an aversion. This may seem too obvious to be worth mentioning, but readers will learn that their taste preferences will change with the transition to a plant based diet. Our senses help us distinguishing between good and bad foods and our senses help protect us from bad foods. Bad foods are not just foods that are bad for you, they are also the foods you just don't want to eat[189].

Food for Thought

1. What determines whether or not a substance is classified as a vitamin? Why is ascorbic acid called Vitamin C?

2. What are the difference between artificial sweeteners, sugar alcohols, novel sweeteners, and natural sweeteners and how are they regulated by the FDA?

3. Acesulfame potassium (or acesulfame-K), TBHQ, and high fructose corn syrup are frequently listed as questionable additives. What are the causes of concern?

4. A Western-type diet, characterized by a significant share of highly processed and refined foods and high content of sugars, salt, fat and protein from red meat, has been recognized as an important factor contributing to the development of metabolic disorders and the obesity epidemic around the world. The Western-type diet is also associated with an increased incidence of chronic kidney disease, and with a chronic inflammatory process that is involved in all stages of atherosclerosis development and is increasingly recognized as a universal mechanism of various chronic degenerative diseases, such as autoimmune diseases, some neoplasms or osteoporosis[190]. What differences would you expect between the Dietary Reference Intakes published by the USDA – 45% - 65% of calories should come from carbohydrate, 10% - 35% of calories should come from protein, 20% - 35% of calories should come from fat – and the actual percentages of macronutrients in the Western-type diet?

Chapter Five: Eat This!

"Then God said, 'I give you every seed-bearing plant on the face of the whole earth and every tree that has fruit with seed in it. They will be yours for food. And to all of the beasts of the earth and all the birds of the air and all the creatures that move on the ground – everything that has the breath of life in it – I give every green plant for food.' And it was so." – Genesis 1

Now that you know how to determine what foods to limit or avoid, let's turn to the question what are the healthful foods? Earlier we said they are foods that provide our essential nutrients, plus energy to sustain growth, health, and life while satiating hunger and reducing the risk of certain disease such as stroke, obesity, cancer, or diabetes. Hence, the key attributes of healthful food are its nutrients, energy content, disease preventive and therapeutic properties, and good taste. The nutrients include the macronutrients – carbohydrates, fats, and proteins – that provide calories and the micronutrients – vitamins and minerals – non-caloric substances that are indirectly involved in energy metabolism. Additionally, phytochemicals are important non-nutritive, non-essential food components believed to be responsible for disease protection or prevention. All vegetables, fruits, and whole foods of every kind possess characteristic arrays of thousands of potentially healthful constituents.

Legal definitions and Guidelines

There also exists legal definitions for references to healthy food products. FDA regulations define *"healthy,"* to mean the product must meet certain criteria that limit the amounts of fat, saturated fat, cholesterol, and sodium, and requires specific minimum amounts of vitamins, minerals, or other beneficial nutrients[191]. The term *"healthy"* and related terms *("health," "healthful," "healthfully," "healthfulness," "healthier," "healthiest," "healthily" and "healthiness"*) may be used only if the food meets certain FDA requirements[192]. And through an indirect characterization the USDA defines healthy foods in its publication *"Healthy Eating Tips."*[193]

There are published guidelines for planning and assessing <u>healthy</u> <u>diets</u>. The Recommended Dietary Allowances (RDAs) are the levels of intake of essential nutrients that, on the basis of scientific knowledge, are judged by the Food and Nutrition Board of the National Research Council to be adequate to meet the known nutrient needs of practically all healthy persons.

There is a safety factor in the RDAs for each nutrient, reflecting the state of knowledge concerning the nutrient, its bioavailability, and variations among the U.S. population. It is intended that the RDAs be both safe and adequate, but not necessarily the highest or lowest figures that the data might justify. RDAs have not been set for all nutrients. Traditionally, RDAs have been established for essential nutrients only when data are sufficient to make reliable recommendations.

The Food and Nutrition Board decided that for planning meals or food supplies, it is technically difficult and biologically unnecessary to design a single day's diet that contains all the RDAs for all the nutrients. Nor, they argue, is there biological reason for expecting that each meal should contain a fixed percentage of an RDA for a nutrient. The RDAs are goals to be achieved over time—at least 3 days for nutrients that turn over rapidly, whereas one or several months might be adequate for more slowly metabolized nutrients. In practice, menus for congregate feeding – e.g. feeding programs such as meals on wheels, food for the elderly – should be designed so that the RDAs are met in a 5- to 10-day rotation.

Note that RDAs should not be confused with Estimated Average Requirements, or EARs. The EAR is used to estimate the RDA. The EAR represents the average daily nutrient intake level estimated to meet the requirement of half of the healthy individuals in a particular life stage or gender group. The RDA represents the average daily nutrient intake level that meets the nutrient requirements of 97% to 98% of healthy individuals in a particular life stage or gender group[194].

The Nutrients

To better understand the nourishing characteristics of healthful foods are, it is useful to briefly review what the nutrients are and why they are important components of a healthful diet: Nutrients are chemical substances in food that provide the energy for your body's metabolic processes and the other organ and systems functions. The macronutrients are carbohydrate, protein, and fat.

Carbohydrates are found in starchy foods like grain and potatoes, fruits, milk, and yogurt. Other foods like vegetables, beans, nuts, seeds and cottage cheese contain carbohydrates, but in lesser amounts.

Carbohydrate provides 4 calories per gram. They are macronutrients that we need in the largest amounts. And they are the body's main source of fuel. Carbohydrates are easily used by the body for energy. All of the tissues and cells in our body can use glucose for energy. Carbohydrates can be stored in the muscles and liver and later used for energy. Carbohydrates are needed for the central nervous system, the kidneys, the brain, and muscles – including the heart to function properly.

Carbohydrates are important in intestinal health and waste elimination. *"Fiber"* refers to types of carbohydrates that our body cannot digest. They pass through the intestinal tract intact and help to move waste out of the body. Foods high in fiber include fruits, vegetables, and whole grain products. Diets high in fiber have been shown to decrease risks for heart disease, obesity, and they help lower cholesterol. Diets that are low in fiber have been postulated to cause diverticulosis and hemorrhoids, and to increase the risk for certain types of cancers such as colon cancer. However, according to the Nutrition Source at Harvard, cohort studies found that fiber intake had very little, if any, link with colon cancer[195].

Choose to eat whole grains – such as oatmeal, whole wheat bread, and brown rice, and avoid highly refined grains that have less fiber and fewer nutrients, vitamins and minerals, antioxidants, and phytochemicals. Avoid starches and refined carbohydrates, eat them only occasionally, in small amounts. Whole wheat, brown rice, quinoa, millet, farro, and amaranth are healthful. There is a useful index (**C/F**) for breads and cereals, which is the ratio of the number of grams per serving of carbohydrates to the number of grams of fiber per serving. Harvard School of Public Health recommends scores of 5 and under (**C/F ≤ 5**) for cereals and 10 and under (**C/F ≤ 10**) for breads.

> ## Grains or Cereals
>
> Grains, also called cereals, are the seeds of plants cultivated for food. When whole, they include the germ, bran, and endosperm.
>
> The *bran* is the layer of the grain that contains fiber, antioxidants, B vitamins, phytochemicals, and 50-80% of minerals in grains like iron, copper, zinc, magnesium.
>
> The *endosperm* is the middle largest layer containing mostly carbohydrates, protein, and small amounts of some B vitamins and minerals.
>
> The *germ* is the inner component containing healthy fats, B vitamins, phytochemicals, and antioxidants like vitamin E.
>
> Refined grains are mainly composed of only the endosperm portion of the grain. The milling process removes most of the bran and some germ, along with the majority of fiber, vitamins, minerals, antioxidants and phytochemicals. As much as 75% of phytochemicals are lost in the refining process.
>
> *Enrichment* is the replacement of certain vitamins and minerals that were removed in processing. However, grain enrichment does not replace many of the health promoting components originally found in whole grains.
>
> Most whole grains are abundant sources of dietary fiber and other nutrients, such as minerals and antioxidants, which have shown beneficial effects on human health including improvement of weight loss, insulin sensitivity, and lipid profile, as well as inhibition of systemic inflammation[196].

Protein is found in meats, poultry, fish, meat substitutes, cheese, milk, nuts, legumes (beans, peas, lentils, soybeans, and peanuts), and in smaller quantities in starchy foods and vegetables.

Protein provides 4 calories per gram. They are needed for growth and development, tissue repair, immune functions, fabricating essential hormones and enzymes, preserving lean muscle mass, and providing energy when carbohydrate is not available.

Protein that comes from animal sources contains all of the essential amino acids that we need. Plant sources of protein, on the other hand, generally do not contain all of the essential amino acids, particularly lysine, tryptophan, methionine, and phenylalanine. Quinoa is one of the exceptions, and has been recognized as a complete food due to its protein quality[197].

> **Quinoa**
>
> Quinoa is not technically a cereal grain, but is a "pseudo-cereal" – food that is cooked and eaten like grains and has a similar nutrient profile. Botanically, quinoa is related to beets, chard, and spinach.
>
> Quinoa is one of the few plant foods that is a complete protein, with all the essential amino acids. It is naturally low in fat and relatively low in calories.
>
> The most common whole-grain foods (breads, baked goods, cereals, pasta and crackers) contain gluten. Quinoa is gluten free.
>
> It is rich source of soluble and insoluble dietary fiber, a good sources of B-complex group of vitamins, vitamin E (a-tocopherol) and essential fatty acids such as linoleic and alpha-linolenic acid and an excellent source of minerals including iron, copper, calcium, potassium, manganese, and magnesium[198].

Soy is a complete protein, which contains all the essential amino acids. Whole soy foods like edamame (green soybeans) or soy nuts provide minerals such as zinc, magnesium, iron, and selenium. Soybeans are by far the most concentrated source of isoflavones in the human diet[199]. Fermented soy products, such as miso, tempeh, and soy yogurt, are probiotic (they contain bacteria which contribute to the health of the intestinal tract).

Plant-based <u>meals</u> that contain all of the essential amino acids are not uncommon. Examples include: brown rice and beans; peanut butter and whole wheat bread; cornbread and pinto beans; refried beans with wheat or corn tortillas; and falafel and whole wheat pita.

Choose to eat proteins from beans (garbanzo, lima, fava, black, kidney, navy, great northern, pinto, adzuki, mung), lentils, seeds, nuts and soybeans (including tempeh and tofu), limit/avoid red meats, and avoid processed meats. If you are not opposed to eating fresh fish and poultry, eat them only occasionally, in small amounts. Harvard includes in its pyramid (discussed below) chicken and turkey as good sources of protein that can be low in saturated fat, and also eggs even though they contain fairly high levels of cholesterol.

Meat Substitutes and Vegan Protein Sources

There are several available alternatives to nearly every type of meat, including chicken-, pork-, fish-, and beef-style products. These healthful substitutes can provide new and familiar savory textures and flavors.

Tofu, Seitan, and Tempeh – Meat Substitutes and Vegan Protein Sources

Tofu, also known as bean curd, is made from soybeans – an excellent source of high quality protein. It is high in protein, low in fat, and cholesterol-free. It also contains phytochemicals, such as isoflavones and soy saponins. Soy isoflavones and saponins are thought to be protective of colon cancer[200].

Tofu absorbs the flavors and marinades it is exposed to. It comes in a wide variety of styles (consistency or texture). Three of the most popular are silken tofu, which is smooth and creamy, can be used in place of cream in soups or as a substitute for mayonnaise or sour cream in salad dressings and dips; soft tofu, which is moist and more firm than silken tofu, can be substituted for soft cheese like ricotta; and firm and extra firm tofu will hold its texture and shape and can be used to substitute for egg dishes, and meats in salads, shish-ka-bobs or fajitas[201].

Tempeh is a soy product made by a natural culturing and controlled fermentation process that binds soybeans into a cake form. It assimilates spices and marinades well like tofu. Tempeh is available in many commercially-prepared varieties, including sprouted, smoked, and with different grain and spice preparations, like flax and barley. The soy carbohydrates in tempeh are more readily available and easily digestible as a result of the fermentation process. Soybeans contain no vitamin B_{12}. The relatively high B_{12} content found in some commercial tempeh has been shown by researchers to be the result of bacterial contamination during production[202]. Tempeh has a nutty flavor that is unlike tofu.

Seitan, or *"wheat gluten,"* has a similar look and texture of meat when cooked. Seitan can be prepared using either whole wheat flour or vital wheat gluten and is made by rinsing away the starch in the wheat, leaving a high-protein gluten behind. Because it is comprised of pure gluten, seitan is protein- and calorie-dense. Seitan is popular in recipes mixing it with beans, grains, tofu, and tempeh to achieve different textures[203].

3 oz. servings	Tofu	Tempeh	Seitan
Calories	70	173	90
Fat (g)	3.5	6	1
Sodium (mg)	20	8	380
Carbs (g)	2	12	3
Fiber (g)	<1	9	1
Protein (g)	8	16.6	18

Fat is found in meat, poultry, nuts, milk products, butters and margarines, oils, lard, fish, grain products and salad dressings.

Fat is the most concentrated source of energy. It provides 9 calories per gram. Fat is needed for normal growth and development, the absorption of certain vitamins (A, D, E, K, and carotenoids), maintaining cell membranes, and cushioning the body's organs. Fat provides taste, consistency, and stability to foods.

Try replacing saturated fat –found in meat products – and trans fat –found in fried and baked goods –in your diet with: 1)polyunsaturated fats including vegetable oils and omega-3 fatty acids – found in fish, seeds and nuts, and canola oil – and 2)with monounsaturated fats – found in avocados and many plant-based oils, such as olive oil and canola oil. Harvard's pyramid, discussed below, includes among good sources of healthy unsaturated fats, soy, corn, sunflower, and peanut oil, plus trans fat–free margarines.

> **Monounsaturated Fat**
>
> Monounsaturated fat is a type of fat is found in avocados, canola oil, nuts, olives and olive oil, and seeds. Eating food that has more monounsaturated fat (or *"healthy fat"*) instead of saturated fat (like butter) may help lower cholesterol and reduce heart disease risk. However, monounsaturated fat has the same number of calories as other types of fat and will contribute to weight gain if you eat too much of it.
>
> **Polyunsaturated Fat**
>
> Polyunsaturated fat is a type of fat that is liquid at room temperature. There are two types of polyunsaturated fatty acids (PUFAs): omega-6 and omega-3. Omega-6 fatty acids are found in liquid vegetable oils, such as corn oil, safflower oil, and soybean oil. Omega-3 fatty acids come from plant sources—including canola oil, flaxseed, soybean oil, and walnuts—and from fish and shellfish.
>
> Omega-3 fatty acid supplements are <u>not</u> recommended for cardiovascular protection, because they have no significant impact on all-cause mortality, acute myocardial infarction, sudden death, or stroke[204]. Additionally, taking potent fish oil supplements has been linked to a 43% increased risk for prostate cancer overall, and a 71% increased risk for aggressive prostate cancer[205].

According to the Dietary Reference Intakes published by the USDA, 45% - 65% of calories should come from carbohydrate, 10% - 35% of calories should come from protein, 20% - 35% of calories should come from fat. The <u>quality</u> of each of those macronutrients is very important.

Micronutrients play a central part in metabolism and in the maintenance of tissue function. Their biochemical functions include acting as <u>cofactors</u> (cofactors are inorganic substances like zinc and selenium required for, or to increase the rate of, catalysis) in metabolism; as <u>coenzymes</u> (coenzymes are organic molecules like vitamins or metabolites of vitamins that are required by certain enzymes to carry out catalysis) in metabolism; as <u>antioxidants</u>; and in genetic control mechanisms, like zinc that binds to DNA and regulates transcription (the process by which the information in a strand of DNA is copied into a new molecule of messenger RNA).

An adequate intake of micronutrients is vital for human function. However, **the prevention or treatment of diseases that are not due to micronutrient deficiency cannot be expected to occur from increased intake. Furthermore, the use of excess supplements may be harmful to people who do not need them.**

You can get an adequate intake of vitamins and minerals from nutrient-dense foods, like leafy greens, dried beans, whole grains, salmon, and colorful vegetables such as broccoli, scallions, and tomatoes.

Phytochemicals

Plant-based foods are complex mixtures of bioactive compounds. Phytochemicals are the bioactive compounds found in plants that are capable of affecting human health. However, they are not required to sustain human life.

A growing body of research suggest that phytochemicals can protect us from a variety of diseases. Phytochemicals present in vegetables and fruits are believed to reduce the risk of several major diseases including cardiovascular diseases, cancers, neurodegenerative disorders, and other diseases. And many chemicals found in edible plants are known to inhibit metastatic progression of cancer[206].

Nevertheless, evidence that these effects are due to specific nutrients or phytochemicals is limited. The knowledge of the potential health effects of individual phytochemicals is derived from information on the health effects of the foods that contain those phytochemicals. Therefore, it is necessary to eat a varied and colorful whole food, plant-based diet in order to accrue the full benefits of phytochemicals. **Nutrient dense vegetables and fruits are a better source of phytochemicals than energy dense foods.**

There are literally thousands of phytochemicals that have been studied and they have classified in various ways. According to one source the major classes of phytochemicals with disease-preventing functions are: dietary fiber, antioxidants, detoxifying agents, immunity-potentiating agents, and neuropharmacological agents. But each class of these functional agents consists of a wide range of chemicals with differing potency. For example, the <u>antioxidant</u> function is exhibited by isothiocyanates, flavonoids, carotenoids, and phenolic compounds[207].

Some phytochemicals have more than one function. For example, certain bioactive components from the plants have been confirmed for their <u>anti-cancer</u> activities. Isothiocyanates (found in broccoli, cauliflower, and Brussel sprouts) may suppress tumor growth and hormone production. Flavonoids (in apples, grapefruit, red wine, etc.), and lycopene (found in tomatoes) also demonstrate protection against cancer[208].

The text box below lists numerous examples of phytochemicals that are reported to have actually been used as cancer chemopreventive and treatment agents.

Phytochemicals as Chemopreventive and Treatment Agents

Numerous examples of phytochemicals are reported to have actually been used as cancer chemopreventive and treatment agents including:

Apigenin from parsley. Apigenin, a flavone present in vegetables such as parsley, celery, chamomile.

Curcumin from turmeric. Curcumin, is the major components of popular Indian spice turmeric, a member of the ginger family.

Crocetin from saffron. Saffron is both a spice and a food colorant.

Cyanidins from grapes. Cyanidin is an extract of pigment from red berries such as grapes, blackberry, cranberry, raspberry, or apples and plums, red cabbage and red onion.

Diindolylmethane (DIM) and Indole-3-carbinol (I3C) from brassica vegetables. I3C is found in brassica vegetables, such as broccoli, cauliflower, collard greens. DIM is a digestion derivative of I3C formed in the acidic environment of the stomach.

Epigallocatechin gallate (EGCG) from green tea. EGCG is the most abundant catechin compounds in green tea.

Fisetin from strawberries, and apples. Fisetin is a flavone found in various plants such as Acacia greggii, Acacia berlandieri, Euroasian smoketree, parrot tree, strawberries, apple, persimmon, grape, onion, and cucumber.

Genistein from soybean. Genistein is an isoflavone that originates from a number of plants such as lupine, fava beans, soybeans, kudzu, and psoralea, Flemingia vestita, and coffee.

Gingerol from gingers. Gingerol is the active component of fresh ginger with distinctive spiciness.

Kaempferol from tea, broccoli, and grapefruit. Kaempferol is a natural flavonol isolated from tea, broccoli, grapefruit, Brussels sprouts, apples, etc.

Lycopene from tomato. Lycopene is a bright red pigment and phytochemical from tomatoes, red carrots, watermelons, and red papayas.

Phenethyl isothiocyanate (PEITC) from cruciferous vegetable such as watercress, broccoli, cabbage, etc.

Resveratrol from grapes. Resveratrol is a natural phenol and can be found in the red grapes skin, peanuts and in other fruits. Note: although resveratrol can inhibit the growth of cancer cells in culture and in some animal models, it is not known whether resveratrol can prevent and/or help treat cancer in humans[209].

Rosmarinic acid from rosemary. Rosmarinic acid is a natural antioxidant found in culinary spice and medicinal herbs – such as lemon balm, peppermint, sage, thyme, oregano, and rosemary – used to treat numerous ailments.

Sulforaphane from cruciferous vegetables. Sulforaphane is an organosulfur compound obtained from cruciferous vegetables such as broccoli, Brussels sprouts and cabbages. The enzyme

> myrosinase in GI tract transforms glucoraphanin into sulforaphane upon damage to the plant such as from chewing. Broccoli sprouts and cauliflower sprouts are rich in glucoraphanin.
>
> <u>Triterpenoids</u> from wax-like coatings of fruits and medicinal herbs. The triterpenoids refers to a group of phytochemicals that have been sub-classified into cucurbitanes, dammaranes, ergostanes, friedelanes, lanostanes, limonoids, lupanes, oleananes, tirucallanes, ursanes – and the list is still growing[210].

Taste and Flavor

At this point the reader should have a good understanding of what makes plant based foods healthful. But for many people some healthful foods may not be tasty and few if any are delicious. The "flav" in flavonoids, which often impart bitter tastes to food, is not a prefix flavorful or an indication of pleasing flavor. You may need to get past objectionable taste sensations like overly bitter, sour, slimy or mushy textures, and visual food textural blocks. Although your tastes will change as you transition to eating the most healthful nutrient dense foods, you may want to explore opportunities to enhance the flavor of foods that are difficult to adapt to. And you will want to discover ways to make boring or objectionable food savory and even delicious without compromising its nutritional values.

Contempt for nutritional value is a hallmark of fad foods. From the ridiculousness of deep-fried zucchini, avocadoes, and other vegetables to the farcical deep-fried pizza, spaghetti and meatballs, and Oreo cookies, there are numerous appetite stimulating schemes that throw out the champagne with the cork. Chain food restaurants commonly don't let nutrition compromise profits from their expensive, salty salads that feature steak, fried chicken, shrimp, and potatoes, crumbled, sliced, or fried cheese, bacon, sugar coated dried cranberries, token nuts or seeds, and full-fat dressings, that can exceed 1,200 calories per serving. And some restaurants counterfeit their menu items of salads and other dishes, by deceptively adorning them with char-marked processed chicken meat instead of genuine grilled chicken.

One of the biggest on-going areas of challenge is the dearth of tasty, healthful low-cal salad dressing, but the most effective solution lies with the clever use of spices. Using spices and herbs (parsley, chives, thyme, sage, oregano, mint, rosemary, tarragon, basil, dill, cilantro, coriander, marjoram, caraway, savory) can enhance the flavor of healthful foods without adding sugar, salt, and calories. And spices and herbs can contribute to satisfying visual food textures and aromas[211]. We cannot overstate the value of spices and herbs. Remember this: *You will harvest great rewards when you harmonize with spices and herbs.*

Some healthful supplements that can further enhance the flavor of salads include: flavored and seasoned vinegars, fresh fruits (strawberries, apples, blueberries, etc.) dried cherries or cranberries, seeds (pumpkin, sunflower, hemp seeds, etc.), nuts (walnuts, almonds, pistachios, etc.), and quinoa. Mashed avocado or hummus toppings can make salads and other dishes come alive. Adding the vegetarian staples tofu, tempeh, or seitan flavored with spices and herbs can provide healthy alternatives to meat and eggs in salads, sandwiches, and other meals.

Fruits and Vegetables

Filling your diet with fruits and vegetables, and meat substitutes creates less room for harmful foods with saturated fat, which has been linked to cardiovascular disease.

The more fruits and vegetables you eat, the less likely you are to develop chronic diseases. Research supports evidence of that inverse relationship of fruit and vegetable consumption with development of chronic disease. In particular, a 2014 review published in the European Journal of Nutrition presented the following findings:

> **Vegetables and Fruit in the Prevention of Chronic Diseases**
>
> 1) For hypertension, coronary heart disease, and stroke, there is convincing evidence that increasing the consumption of vegetables and fruit reduces the risk of disease.
>
> 2) There is probable evidence that the risk of cancer in general is inversely associated with the consumption of vegetables and fruit.
>
> 3) In addition, there is possible evidence that an increased consumption of vegetables and fruit may prevent body weight gain. As overweight is the most important risk factor for type 2 diabetes mellitus, an increased consumption of vegetables and fruit therefore might indirectly reduces the incidence of type 2 diabetes mellitus. Independent of overweight, there is probable evidence that there is no influence of increased consumption on the risk of type 2 diabetes mellitus.
>
> 4) There is possible evidence that increasing the consumption of vegetables and fruit lowers the risk of certain eye diseases, dementia and the risk of osteoporosis.
>
> 5) Likewise, current data on asthma, chronic obstructive pulmonary disease, and rheumatoid arthritis indicate that an increase in vegetable and fruit consumption may contribute to the prevention of these diseases[212].

Produce is worthy of due respect, but don't expect miracles. The adage *"An apple a day keeps the doctor away"* is good advice but it's not to be taken literally. Proverb-busting research has found daily apple eaters had just as many doctor visits as those who ate fewer or no apples[213].

However, in numerous epidemiological studies, apples have been associated with a decreased risk of chronic diseases such as cardiovascular disease, cancer, and asthma. *In vitro* and animal studies have demonstrated that apples have high antioxidant activity, can inhibit cancer cell proliferation, decrease lipid oxidation, and lower cholesterol, potentially explaining their role in reducing risk of chronic disease. Apples contain a wide variety of phytochemicals, many of which have been found to have strong antioxidant activity and anticancer activity[214].

This digression on apples is not to imply that apples are the most healthful fruits. It is just one of the many excellent foods that are commonly available. Indeed, apples with and ANDI score of 53 are presumably less than half as nutritious as blueberries with an ANDI of 132[215].

Experts believe that increased consumption of fruits and vegetables promotes cardiovascular health and reduced risk of diabetes. But it is interesting to note that a recent study concluded evidence to date suggests that *"a broad effort to increase consumption of fruits and vegetables will not have a major effect on cancer incidence."* [216]

Food Pyramids

There appears to be agreement among nutrition experts on the food groups in healthy plant based diets but there are considerable differences concerning the importance and range of servings for each food group. Food pyramids are simple messages on healthy eating aimed at the general public. Food plates are touted as an improvement over the food pyramid concept because plates are supposedly easier for non-readers to understand. The plate became the new USDA icon following criticism by the food industry and others of its original USDA food pyramid and revisions that followed. The USDA's pyramids were criticized by nutritionists for being too heavily influenced by the meat and dairy industries and scientifically outdated. Others attacked the pyramids for being vague and confusing. The distaste for the USDA pyramid's geometry echoed the sentiment expressed in Antigone by Sophocles: *"No one loves the messenger who brings bad news."*

There are several well known food pyramids (and plates) that are supposed to suggests the types and frequencies of foods that should be enjoyed for health. Nine examples are presented below including: Harvard's Healthy Eating Pyramid, Dr. Joel Fuhrman's Nutritarian Pyramid, the University of Michigan's Integrative Medicine's Healing Foods Pyramid, the Ray Kurzwell and Terry Grossman Transcend Pyramid, the Mayo Clinic Healthy Weight Pyramid, the Loma Linda University Vegetarian Food Pyramid, the Oldways Vegetarian and Vegan Diet Pyramid, Dr. Weil's Anti-Inflammatory Food Pyramid, and the FINUT pyramid.

Food pyramids give a proportional representation as to the volume (by servings, or calories, or daily/weekly) of food from each of the various food groups a person should aim to eat, starting at the base that represents the majority of food to be eaten and progressing to the apex with the smallest area containing foods to be consumed sparingly.

Harvard's Healthy Eating Pyramid

The Harvard pyramid was created as an alternative to USDA's new MyPlate icon, which was recognized as an improvement over the old Food Guide Pyramid and MyPyramid, but still fell short of meeting the expectations of faculty at the Harvard School of Public Health for providing people with the nutrition advice needed to choose the healthiest diets. The Harvard <u>Nutrition Source</u> remarked *"If the only goal of the USDA's food icons is to give us the best possible advice for healthy eating, then they should be grounded in the evidence and be independent of commercial interests."* Harvard's Healthy Eating Pyramid and the Healthy Eating Plate are intended to be based on the best available scientific evidence about the links between diet and health. They attempt to fix fundamental flaws in the USDA food pyramids and plate and offer sound information to help people make better choices about what to eat.

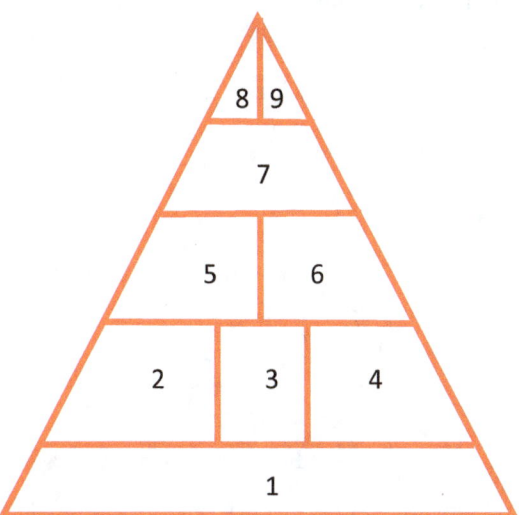

Harvard's Healthy Eating Pyramid

The base of Harvard's 5-tier pyramid (1) is occupied by daily exercise and weight control. This may be meant to underscore the need to address an active healthy lifestyle, not just healthy eating.

The next tier up from the base is a trapezoid divided into three compartments: with vegetables (excluding potatoes) and fruits at one end (2), healthy fats/oils in the middle (3), and whole grains at the opposite end (4). Healthy fats/oils occupy only about 63% as much area as either of the two adjacent trapezoids. In other words, 24% is devoted to healthy fats/oil, and 38% each to vegetables and fruits and to whole grains.

The third tier is comprised of two compartments of equal area: nuts, seeds, beans and tofu on one side (5) and fish, poultry and eggs and the other side (6). The area of the third tier is less than the second tier but greater than the fourth tier.

The fourth tier (7) is occupied by dairy or vitamin D or calcium supplements, and the pinnacle of the pyramid is represented by two equilateral right triangles, one representing red meat, processed meat and butter (8); and the other (9) by potatoes, sugary drinks and sweets, salt and refined grains including white rice, bread and pasta. Harvard's faculty advises: *"If you don't like dairy products, taking a vitamin D and calcium supplement (or taking the right multivitamin) offers an easy and inexpensive way to meet your needs for these micronutrients."* And they suggest switching to fish or chicken (or nuts or beans) in place of red meat and processed meat and switching from butter to olive oil to improve cholesterol levels and lower the risk of heart diseases and diabetes[217].

Dr. Fuhrman's Nutritarian Pyramid

Dr. Fuhrman's Nutritarian Pyramid also addresses fundamental flaws in the USDA's new MyPlate. Dr. Fuhrman's Nutritarian Pyramid is a 5-tier pyramid with low-calorie, nutrient dense foods at the base of the pyramid, and high-calorie, nutrient poor foods are at the apex. As nutrient density decreases, the quantity of foods consumed in the diet also decreases.

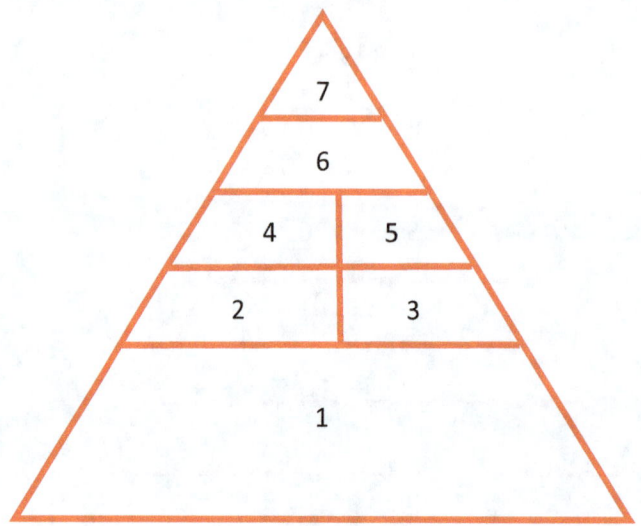

Dr. Fuhrman's Nutritarian Pyramid

As illustrated the pyramid begins at the base (1) with equal shares of raw and cooked vegetables, which may comprise 30-60% of the calories. Fruits (10-40% of calories) occupy one half of the second tier (2) with beans/legumes (10-40% of calories (3)), the third tier is divided equally between seeds, nuts, and avocados (10-40% of calories) on one side (4) and whole grains and potatoes (20% or less of calories) on the other side (5). These three tiers are supposed to comprise 90% of the daily diet.

The area allocations for the last two tiers may not be not entirely clear. According to the description *"If desired, the remaining 10% of the diet may include minimally processed foods such as tortillas, coarsely-ground or sprouted whole grain breads or cereals, tofu, tempeh and a limited amount of animal products, preferably not more than 5 percent of total caloric intake."* However the figure shows eggs, fish, and fat-free dairy (less than 10% of calories) occupying the fourth tier (6). And the pinnacle (7) is reserved for beef, sweets, cheese and processed foods, to be eaten rarely. When the pyramid is viewed together with Dr. Fuhrman's *"Nutritarian Food Plate,"* the presentation is easier to follow.

Nutrient density plays an important role in Dr. Fuhrman's diet plan. As previously mentioned, the Aggregate Nutrient Density Index (ANDI) ranks the nutrient value of whole foods on the basis of how many nutrients they deliver for each calorie consumed. Foods are ranked on a scale of 1-1000 with the most nutrient-dense cruciferous leafy green vegetables scoring 1000. Dr. Fuhrman advises people to consume mostly foods that have an ANDI score greater than 100, but he also recommends eating an adequate assortment of lower ranked plant foods to obtain the full range of human requirements.

According to Dr. Fuhrman, ninety percent of the daily diet should be made up of nutrient rich plant foods, whose calories are accompanied by health-promoting phytochemicals: green and other non-starchy vegetables; fresh fruits; beans and legumes; raw nuts, seeds, and avocados; starchy vegetables; and whole grains[218]. He suggests eating greens, beans, onions, mushrooms, berries, and seeds every day because of their powerful anti-cancer and anti-fat storage effects. And Dr. Fuhrman recommends that people consume greens, beans, onions, mushrooms, berries, seeds and tomatoes on a regular basis to maximize immune function and protection against cancer[219].

University of Michigan Integrative Medicine's Healing Foods Pyramid

The Integrative Medicine's Healing Foods Pyramid is a 10-tier pyramid that emphasizes foods known to have healing benefits. It can provide plant-based food choices with variety and balance, support of a healthful environment, and mindful eating. All of the tiers appear to be equal in height.

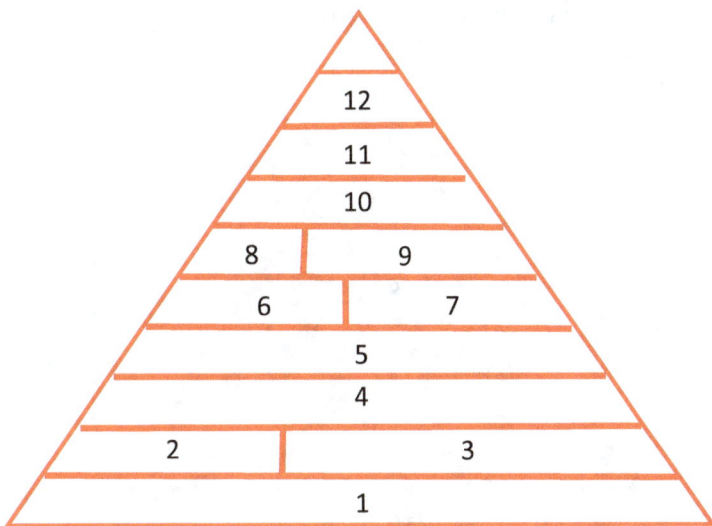

University of Michigan Integrative Medicine's Healing Foods Pyramid

The base tier (1) represents a foundation of water to promote body hydration. The recommended daily water requirements are 9 glasses daily for women and 12 glasses for men, to be consumed in addition to the water in their food. The second tier is shared by fruits (~38 (2)) and vegetables (~62% (3)). The third tier (4) is devoted entirely to whole grains, and legumes occupy the forth tier (5). Healthy fats (52.3% (6)) and seasonings (47.7% (7)) such as herbs, onions, and garlic) share the fifth tier. The sixth tier is comprised of eggs (33.5% (8)) and dairy (66.5% (9)), and the seventh tier (10) consists only of fish and seafood. The eight tier (11) is devoted entirely to lean meats. The ninth tier (12) is for *"accompaniments"* including alcohol, dark chocolate and tea. The pinnacle is empty, reserved for the user's addition of food healing to that individual, to be consumed occasionally, thus personalizing each pyramid.

The Healing Foods Pyramid is designed to offers daily, weekly and optional choices that can be mixed and matched to accommodate most people, whether they are free of health challenges, vegetarian or have specific dietary needs. In the interactive, web-based version, a click on a category immediately takes the user to Facts About guidelines that specify serving sizes, the recommended frequency to eat the foods or drink the beverages, information about the health benefits and concerns of each of the categories[220,221].

Transcend Pyramid by Ray Kurzweil and Terry Grossman

Ray Kurzweil and Terry Grossman published a 5- to 6-tier (one of the tiers has two levels) pyramid that attempted to refine the Harvard Pyramid, which they criticized for its emphasis on grains, due to the higher glycemic loads of whole grains (and fruits) compared to vegetables. And they criticized Harvard's emphasis on vegetable oils, and the inclusion of high fat dairy products, which should be avoided. They also pointed to the failure to distinguish between healthy (e.g. extra-virgin olive oil) and unhealthy oils, and not recognizing the distinction between fish high in omega-3 fats and less desirable sources of proteins such as poultry and eggs.

Their *"Transcend"* pyramid emphasizes low glycemic-load vegetables, healthy fats, such as avocados, nuts and seeds, lean animal protein, fish, and extra virgin olive oil.

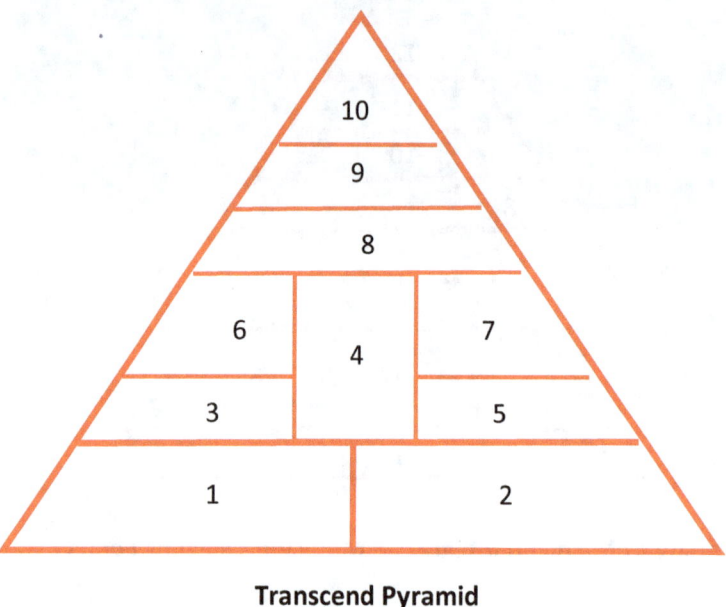

Transcend Pyramid

The first tier at the base of the pyramid is divided equally between vegetables (mostly green above ground (1)) with 5-7 daily servings, and water and green tea (1-5 cups (2)).

The second tier has five compartments. It is a trapezoid that contains two pairs of stacked trapezoids that surround a columnar rectangle. Fish (0-2 servings) in a lower left trapezoid (3) and low-fat dairy foods plus egg whites (0-2 servings) in a lower right trapezoid (5) each occupy approximately 16.8% of the tier. The columnar rectangle (4) is a middle compartment that separates the two pairs of stacked trapezoids on each side. The middle compartment is labeled vegetable protein (soy products, miso, tempeh, tofu) with 2-4 servings and its share of the tier space is about 24.4%. The upper left trapezoid (6) has low GL carbs (beans, lentils, whole grains) with 2-3 servings. Its share of the second tier space is approximately 21%, equal to the upper right trapezoid (7), which is occupied by lean meats (skinless poultry, lean beef) with 0-1 servings.

The third tier (8) is labeled healthy fats, including nuts, seeds, extra-virgin olive oil, avocado, fish oil with 0-3 daily servings. The fourth tier (9) is for fruits, mostly low glycemic load melons, berries, with 0-3 servings, and the top tier (10) is labeled supplements, red wine[222].

Mayo Clinic Healthy Weight Pyramid

The Mayo Clinic Healthy Weight Pyramid is a 5-tier pyramid that was designed as a tool to help people lose weight or maintain their weigh. The pyramid is based on choosing foods with low energy density (few calories for their bulk), which allows you to consume fewer calories while still eating the same amount of food you're accustomed to making you feel full.

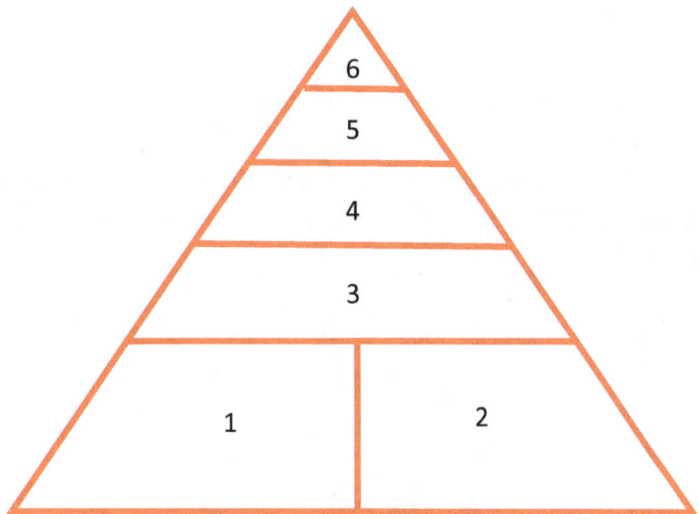

Mayo Clinic Healthy Weight Pyramid

The first tier at the base of the pyramid is divided equally between fruits (unlimited consumption but with a minimum of 3 servings daily (1)) and vegetables (unlimited consumption but with a minimum of 4 servings daily (2)). Whole fresh, frozen and canned fruits without added sugar are recommended, but fruit juices and dried fruits are to be limited. Fresh vegetables are preferred but frozen or canned without added fat or salt are also OK. More dark green, red and orange varieties are encouraged. Starchy, higher calorie vegetables such as corn and potatoes count as carbohydrates.

The second tier (3) is for carbohydrates at 4 to 8 daily servings, followed by protein/dairy in the third tier (4) with 3 to 7 daily servings.

The carbohydrates group consists mostly of grains or food made from grains. Whole grains are preferred, including for example whole-grain cereal, whole-wheat bread, whole-wheat pasta, oatmeal and brown rice.

The best choices of protein and dairy are low in fat and calories, such as fish, skinless white-meat poultry, fat-free dairy foods, egg whites and legumes (lentils, beans and peas).

The forth tier (5) is labeled fats, with an allowance for 3 to 5 daily servings, and the pinnacle (6) is for sweets at up to 75 calories per day.

Good fats, such as olive oil, avocado, nuts, nut butters, etc. are recommended, but saturated fats and trans fats are to be avoided.

The examples in the sweets group include candies, cakes, cookies, pies, doughnuts, and other desserts, as well as table sugar.

Daily physical activity is recommended.[223]

Oldways Vegetarian and Vegan Diet Pyramid

Oldways is a nonprofit food and nutrition education organization[224].

Oldways, the Harvard School of Public Health, and the European Office of the World Health Organization introduced the classic Mediterranean Diet in 1993 at a conference in Cambridge, MA, along with a Mediterranean Diet Pyramid[225,226].

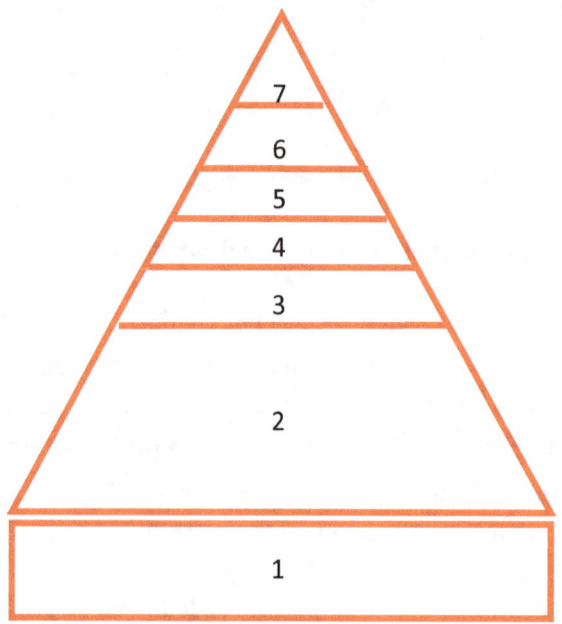

Oldways Vegetarian and Vegan Diet Pyramid

Mediterranean diets remain popular because they are not low fat diets, easy to adopt, and stick to. Note, however, there are a variety of diet styles within the Mediterranean diet and the heavy use of olive oil is problematic.

The Oldways Vegetarian and Vegan Diet Pyramid was created in collaboration with a committee of doctors and nutritionists from the Harvard School of Public Health, Brigham and Women's Hospital, and Loma Linda University, among other renowned institutions, and was presented in October 2013 at the Academy of Nutrition and Dietetics' Food & Nutrition Conference in Houston.

The 6-tier pyramid that rests upon a foundation of physical activity (1).

The base of the pyramid (2) is comprised of fruits and vegetables. The second tier (3) is for whole grains including rice, barley, millet, oats, quinoa, bread, cereal, and pasta.

The third tier (4) is occupied by beans, peas, lentils, and soy. The fourth tier (5) is for nuts, peanuts, seeds, peanut/nut butters.

The fifth tier (6) is labeled herbs, spices, and plant oils. Finally, the apex (7) is reserved for options for vegetarians: eggs and/or dairy including yogurt, cheese, and cottage cheese.

The next pyramid is of historical interest. It was published in 1997. Note that it does not place vegetables at the base level.

Loma Linda University Vegetarian Food Pyramid

The Loma Linda University Vegetarian Food Pyramid is a 6-tier pyramid. At the base are two trapezoids. The larger one, which occupies about 2/3rd, is for whole grains (5-12 daily servings (1)). Legumes and soy (1-3 daily servings (2)) are in the adjacent compartment.

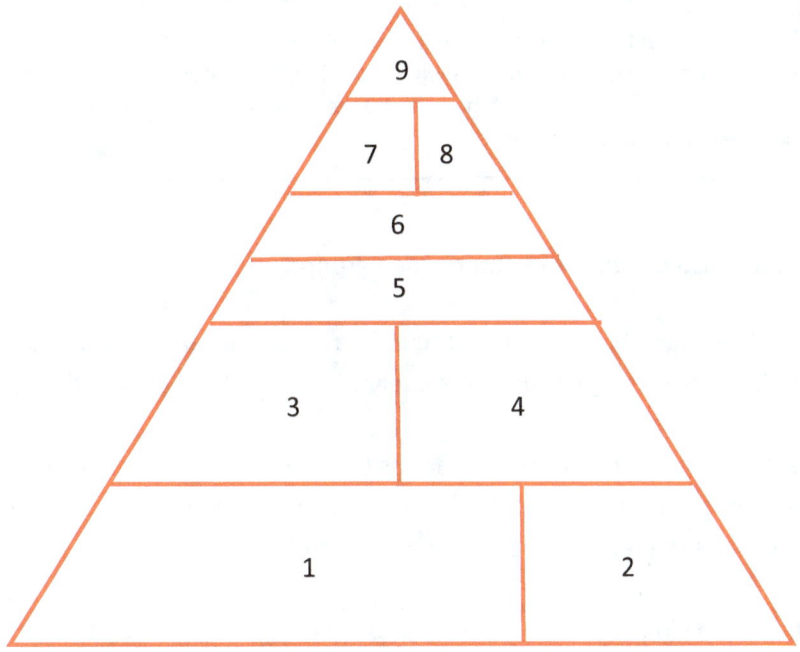

Loma Linda University Vegetarian Food Pyramid

The second tier is shared equally by fruits (3-4 daily servings (3)), and vegetables (6-9 daily servings (4)). Together the first and second tier comprise more than half of the area of the pyramid.

Nuts and seeds (1-2 daily servings) make up the third tier (5), followed by vegetable oils (0-2 daily servings) on the fourth level (6).

The fifth tier contains dairy (0-2 daily servings (7)) and eggs (0-1 daily servings (8)). The area of the eggs trapezoid appears to be 40% of the tier compared to dairy at 60%.

The pinnacle (9) is reserved for sweets.

The pyramid is accompanied by a table that lists the recommended daily servings for vegan and for lacto-ovo diets – diets that exclude meat, fish and poultry, but allow dairy products and eggs.

Exercise, adequate water intake, and exposure to sunlight are included as recommended life style habits[227].

Dr. Weil's Anti-Inflammatory Food Pyramid

Dr. Weil's Anti-Inflammatory Food Pyramid is a twelve-tier food pyramid with 15 categories. For each category, information is provided about serving amounts, sizes, and *"healthy choices."* An example of the additional information is presented in the text box shown below for Healthy Sweets, the category that occupies the top level of the pyramid[228].

> **HEALTHY SWEETS**
> **How much:** Sparingly
> **Healthy choices:** Unsweetened dried fruit, dark chocolate, fruit sorbet
> **Why**: Dark chocolate provides polyphenols with antioxidant activity. Choose dark chocolate with at least 70 percent pure cocoa and have an ounce a few times a week. Fruit sorbet is a better option than other frozen desserts.

Water is the 16th category listed with the recommended groups.

The base level is shared by Vegetables (1), which occupies a hexagonal area of about 59.3% and Fruits (2) at 40.7%. Fruits and Vegetables comprise approximately 29% of the total area of the pyramid.

The second level is split among Whole & Cracked Grains (3), in a hexagonal area of about 41.5% of the total area of that level, next to Pasta *al dete* (4) in a rectangle with a share of about 25.7%, and Beans & Legumes (5), which occupies the remaining 32.8% of the area of the second level.

Healthy Fats, including extra virgin olive oil, expeller-pressed canola oil, nuts, and seeds are on the third level (6). Fish & Seafood (7), such as wild Alaskan salmon, Alaskan black cod, and sardines occupy the forth level, which is enclosed in an area of approximately 9.3% of the total area of the pyramid.

Dr. Weil's Anti-Inflammatory Food Pyramid

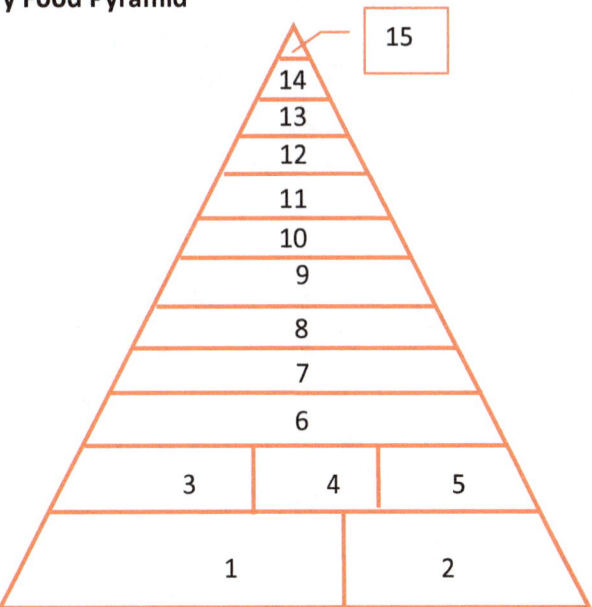

The fifth level is devoted to Whole Soy Foods (8), the sixth level reserved for Cooked Asian Mushrooms (9), and the seventh level is labeled Other Sources of Protein (10) – high quality natural cheeses and yogurt, omega-3 enriched eggs, skinless poultry, and lean meats. The area in seventh level is about 5.2% of the total area of the pyramid.

The eighth level is for Healthy Herbs & Spices (11), followed by Tea (12) on level nine, Supplements (13) on level ten, and Red Wine (14) on level eleven. The top level of the pyramid is labeled Healthy Sweets (15), which are to be consumed sparingly.

Food pyramids are popular in many countries throughout the world[229]. Designs for dietary pyramids are continuing to evolve, including pyramids with more than one dimension, designed to promote healthful eating and active healthy lifestyles. For example, the Iberoamerican Nutrition Foundation (FINUT) pyramid of healthy lifestyles is a tetrahedron, with three lateral faces corresponding to the facets of food and nutrition, physical activity and rest, and education and hygiene.

The **FINUT Pyramid** is similar to the Mediterranean diet pyramid and is not recommended but included here simply because it illustrates a pyramid with multiple faces. Each lateral face is divided into two triangles. The food and nutrition face includes a 7-tier pyramid with water and drinks at the base (1). The following six tiers are labeled *"consume daily."*

Cereals and cereal products (greater than 50% whole grain) are on the second level (2), followed by fruits and vegetables and related products on the third tier (3).

Milk and dairy products, particularly fermented milks and cheese occupy the fourth level (4), which is below olive and other healthy oils on the fifth tier (5). Healthy unsaturated oils include rapeseed or colza, canola, sunflower and soybean oils for use in salads, cooking, and frying.

The sixth level (6) includes poultry and other white meats, eggs, fish and seafood, and pulses (beans, lentils, peas) and nuts. And the pinnacle (7) is occupied by cakes/sweets, red meat, and animal fats, or high-fat products, which are grouped to be *"consumed occasionally."*

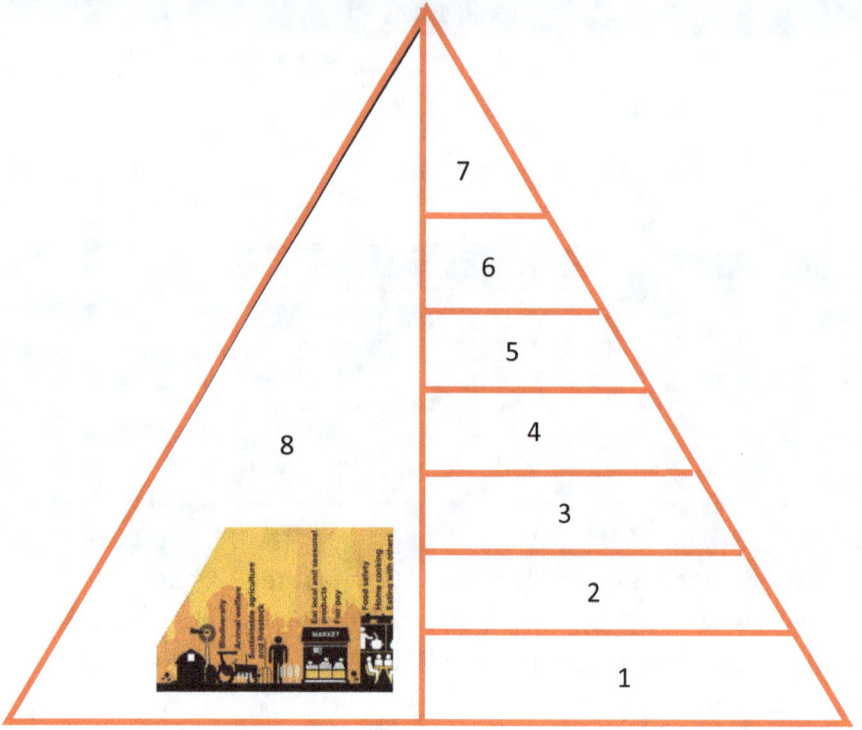

FINUT PYRAMID

There is a triangle (8) adjacent to the food and nutrition face, described above, with several pictograms – descriptive symbols – aimed at emphasizing good food habits and behaviors favoring environmental sustainability and healthy living. This is shown in the insert below.

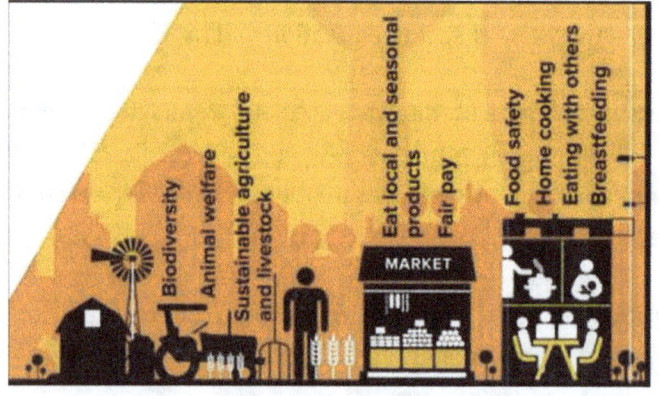

FINUT PICTOGRAMS

Scanning right to left, the first pictogram shows a familial setting that emphasizes the importance of breastfeeding to sustain healthy growth and development. Other elements of the pictogram are eating with others (particularly with family), cooking at home, and food safety, which presumably leads to varied and slow eating with relatively small portions.

The next pictogram labeled market is meant to recommend fair pay, eating of local and seasonal products.

A pictogram with the label sustainable agriculture and livestock is focused on food production linked to the environment and socially centered on the ecologic sustainability of the production systems.

The message of an animal welfare pictogram is presumably the avoidance of pesticides to maintain the soil quality and a healthy agrosystems.

The last pictogram labeled biodiversity emphasizes the need to maintain biodiversity as a world heritage for present and future generations[230].

Except for the FINUT pyramid, which is based on the Mediterranean diet, all of the pyramids that we discussed ranked vegetables at the base or in the second tier (8 out of 9). Fruits were most often ranked in the second tier (4 of 9) but also ranked at the base with vegetables (3 of 9), and would have been ranked with vegetables at the base more than half of the time (5 of 9), if two of the pyramids had not included non-food items (exercise, water) in the base. Hence, the message is clear: vegetables and fruits are the regarded as the highest priority foods for plant based diets.

Creating a Personal Pyramid

Readers may wish to use one or more of the published food pyramids and information concerning the nutrient density of foods they eat to construct their own annotated food pyramids for use in planning their meals. Additionally, you might want to attach a pyramid, like the one illustrated on the next page, to the refrigerator door to use as an aid for compiling a shopping list.

This pyramid, which we named **The Toothsome Triangle**, includes a lenticular cloud or halo above the vertex with spices and herbs that allows you to create meals that are full of flavor, delicious and tasty. And the base floats on water, to emphasize the importance of this essential nutrient.

Ninety percent of the daily caloric intake should come from the lower three tiers of the pyramid. And plan to eat more foods with high nutrient density scores and less with low scores.

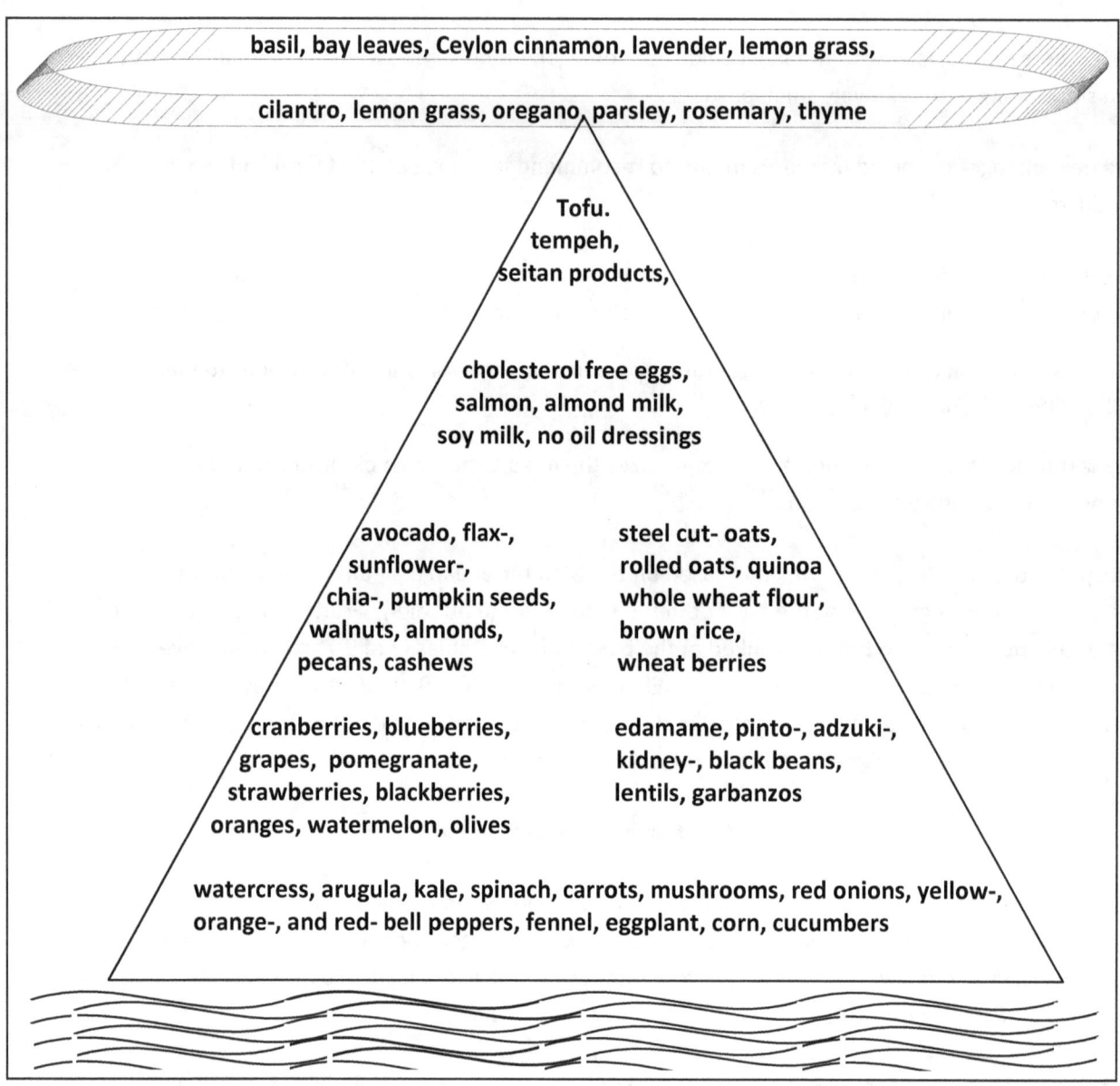

Food for Thought

1. Which of these two opposing statements suggests a healthful diet?

A) *"It is the position of the American Dietetic Association that all foods can fit into a healthful eating style. The ADA strives to communicate healthful eating messages to the public that emphasize the total diet, or overall pattern of food eaten, rather than any one food or meal. If consumed in moderation with appropriate portion size and combined with regular physical activity, all foods can fit into a healthful diet. ..The value of a food should be determined within the context of the total diet because classifying foods as "good" or "bad" may foster unhealthy eating behaviors."*[231]

B) *"Of course there's such a thing as a bad food. At least there is if "bad" is defined on the basis of health. In a sense, a bad food is one whose risks outweigh its nutritional benefits when consumed regularly. And while there is certainly room for disagreement over what should or shouldn't be considered bad, some foods are pretty straightforward. Take lollipops for example….I don't think sugar-coating the fact that *there are indeed bad foods is useful given the numerous diet-related chronic diseases that plague modern-day society. Yet that's exactly what the "no such thing as a bad food" spin does: It takes the sting out of the choice."*

"Truthfully, there are many bad foods that I desperately enjoy. I honestly think I could happily eat potato chips, chicken wings, and nachos each and every meal until the day I die. The thing is, I'd likely die a younger man too, and dying young isn't exactly part of my bucket list." [232]

2. Create a shopping list that emphasizes nutrient density.

3. There is no single ideal Mediterranean diet. There are 18 countries with coasts on the Mediterranean sea. Food habits in Mediterranean countries vary among those countries and were different 20 or 30 years ago, as they were recovering from the Second World War, than they are today. Show how energy density can be used to rank the healthful quality of Mediterranean diets?

Chapter Six: Tools and Aids

"There is a great satisfaction in building good tools for other people to use." – Freeman Dyson

This book was written to aid readers halt their unhealthy eating habits, arrest their desires for irresistible unhealthful foods, and transition to a healthful, high quality plant based lifestyle. This chapter provides a recap of the key take aways, furnishes additional suggestions, and identifies some devices that may facilitate your journey to healthful delicious eating experiences. The information presented here should help you to construct shopping lists for nutritious meals.

Ancient mariners had to rely on dead reckoning (after "deduced rekconing"), the only tool that was available for navigation. Marine navigation has since been automated with instrumentation enabling gigantic vessels to slip in and out of busy harbors aided by tugboats. Likewise, a number of devices are available to aid you on your journey but there will be times when you will have to depend on your skills at deduction.

As a matter of fact, dead reckoning was the first method used in marine navigation that relied on the use of a daily log. A log book is a good item to put on your shopping list. It can be useful to keep a daily record of your diet and exercise, notes about shopping, cooking, dining out, spending, health, and your progress.

Some other useful aids were identified in earlier chapters: In the first chapter we discussed the controversial nature of the literature of nutrition and recommend that you hone your skills at critical reading by consulting the references in Chapter Ten, where there are links (specifically under the heading "Chapter One,") to articles that provide guidance for critically reviewing nutrition studies, evaluating the underpinning evidence, identifying unresolved questions, and understanding the standards for evidence-based recommendations. Chapter Nine includes a number of incisive questions to ask about food and health claims and announcements to help you determine their credibility and how important the results are for you personally.

Daily weight monitoring can provide useful data to help better understand how your dietary intake is affecting your weight and possibly to influence your consumption. In Table 1 we presented an example of a spreadsheet graph of body weight recorded daily each month.

Recall that devices for measuring and tracking body fat were found to be inaccurate and imprecise and therefore inadequate. Instead, we recommended the use of an accurate scale, a tape measure, and a mirror to monitor your weight loss progress. You may want to add a camera to that list of tools. Review articles written for consumers interested in personal scales and cameras are readily available on the Internet.

We know that the storage fat that is of most concern is the visceral fat that surrounds your internal organs and the subcutaneous component of abdominal fat. There are no accurate, practical devices for detection and monitoring central obesity. While we await a modern high tech solution, we have to rely on low tech improvisations like measuring tape, which requires some skill for accurate usage, but is a lot easier to use than devices like skin fold calipers.

Readers who are not satisfied with the precision of measuring their abdominal girth using a tape measure might want to consider fashioning their own device with inspiration from the concept embodied in an old invention, a simple device to permit the accurate and expeditious measurement at the waistline and a region six inches below it. The *"skirt measure"* is illustrated in the following figure.

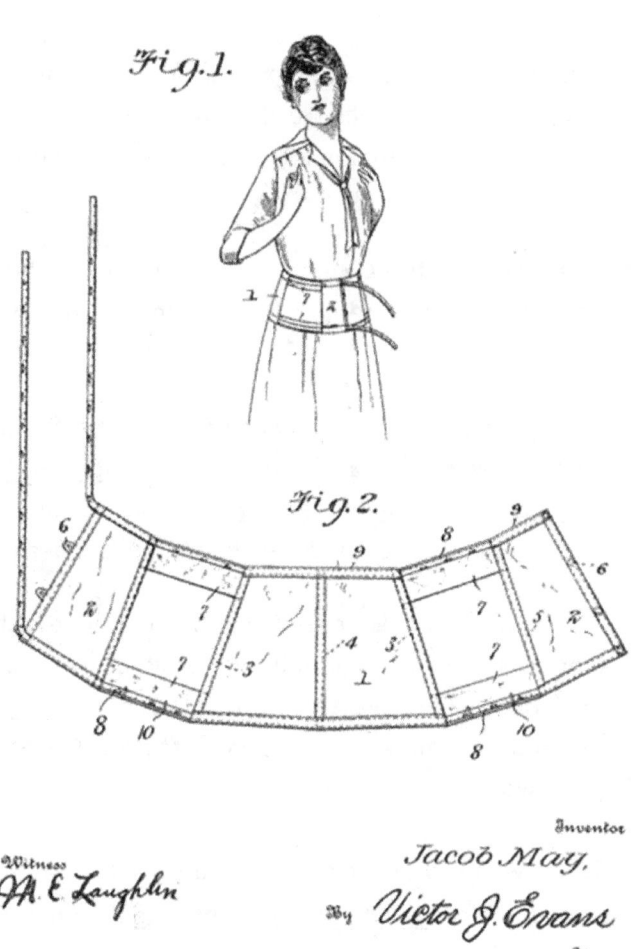

The inventor's explanation of the *"skirt measure."*

"Experience has demonstrated that it is unsatisfactory to the average woman to order a skirt from any of the mail-order houses who make a specialty of supplying women's garments upon measurements furnished them by the customer. There is a region in every skirt which, in the mind of women, must fit with the same degree of precision as the waist band. This region is located six inches below the waist line of the body or waist band of the skirt. Dressmakers or tailors in measuring women have found it extremely difficult to get the exact measurements of the aforesaid region and this is by reason of the fact that a slight slanting or misplacement of the tape during the measuring operation will result in a wrong measurement being had and an improper fit obtained when the cloth is cut to the imperfect measurement. When an imperfect fit is had in the aforesaid region, what is known as the general line of the skirt, has to be altered in order to effect correction.

It is the object of the present invention to overcome this objection by providing a simple device which may be readily used to take the proper measure at the waist line and at the region six inches below the said line, and more especially to permit women using the device to take their own measurements as expeditiously and accurately as if done by others."[233]

There are commercially available body circumference measuring devices that are supposed to enable accurate use by a single person, and digital versions are also available for less than $10. However, there seems to be some accuracy and quality issues that need to be addressed before low cost reliable devices are available.

The importance of accurate information is strongly emphasized in this book. Prior to foraging for healthy foods you should seek accurate information concerning the nutrient and energy content of food products from various sources.

Earlier (Chapter Three) we learned that food labels often do not provide sufficient information for a reliable, comprehensive analysis. However, the careful use of the Nutrition Facts labels, augmented by detailed nutrient information that can be found on the Internet could provide sufficient information about the nutrients and caloric values in your foods to help you formulate healthful diets.

Despite the challenges associated with the implementation of the nutrient density concept, we recommended selecting food options based on their nutrient density scores in order to determine the relative nutrient content of the foods that are available to you. Lists of nutrient density scores that can be found on the Internet, in books, and supermarkets. Some links are provided in the references in Chapter Ten under the heading "Chapter Two."

We encouraged ambitious readers with knowledge of elementary algebra and access to Microsoft Excel or other spreadsheet software to try to create a program to optimize their nutrient dense diets. We provided a link to computer code, which could serve as the computational engine by performing the linear programming. The project will require building the interfaces that collect the input and display the results, which can be done with the spreadsheet software. For skilled programmers with an entrepreneurial spirit we suggest creating an app that lists nutrient density scores for foods and an app that designs nutritionally optimal meals from available foods.

In 2003, a FDA Commissioner speaking at the Harvard School of Public Health said, *"People shouldn't need a calculator or an advanced degree in math or nutrition to calculate what makes a healthy diet."*[234] Today we can say that **some** people with a calculator or an advanced degree in math or nutrition can calculate what makes a healthy diet and **most people** will not need a calculator or an advanced degree in math or nutrition to design nutritionally optimal meals from available foods **if and when** a Smart App with that capability becomes available.

Readers may wish to use one or more of the published food pyramids discussed in Chapter Five or use published values for the nutrient density of foods they eat to build and populate their food pyramids for use in planning their meals. We do not recommend using the USDA food pyramid or *"MyPlate."* As noted by Harvard's Nutrition Source, *"The U.S. Department of Agriculture's MyPlate, though it has been revised to reflect some key findings, still doesn't offer the most complete picture when it comes to basic nutrition advice."*[235]

Useful gadgets and appliances

You will need to ask a lot of questions and use your observation skills when shopping for various useful gadgets and appliances including, for example, a kitchen scale with tare function, high speed blender, food processor, mandolin slicer, sharp knives and a knife sharpener, baking pans, a wok, and other utensils. And, possibly a larger refrigerator or a freezer.

A kitchen scale can be used to convert the weight of food items into volumes, e.g. given that one ounce of walnuts contains about x calories, note the volume (about $1/y$ cup), so you don't have to keep weighing serving size portions of nuts, seeds, berries, etc.

A hand-held calculator is useful for shopping if you don't have or prefer not to use a smart phone. Access to the Internet is essential to finding product reviews, competing price options, recipes, and nutritional science information at various links found in this book.

A large binder with tabs can be useful to store recipes that you find online or elsewhere, and a small notebook stored beside your personal scale might be handy to record your weight before entering it into the spreadsheet.

It might be helpful to program your cell phone or a hand-held calculator to convert common units of measure: grams, ounces, pounds, etc. That will be handy when comparison price shopping at supermarkets that use different units (price each vs. price per lb. or unit prices in oz. etc.).
As noted above, you may want to use a computer with a spreadsheet program like Excel to build a spreadsheet to monitor body weight, but you can also track other measures as well.

To better prepare for your trips to the market, make a list of the food additives to avoid compiled from articles you have read, see e.g. the link in endnote 236 in the References.[236] And use the information from the posters in Chapter Three that show nutrition information for the 20 most frequently consumed raw fruits, vegetables, and fish in the United States, to estimate the quantities to purchase based on the nutrients per typical serving sizes.

During the hot summer months it might be a good idea to bring insulated bag(s) when shopping for food and even bags loaded with ice from your freezer or purchased at grocery stores to preserve frozen and perishable food while you are shopping.

Think about useful gadgets and aids that are not yet commercially available; chances are if there is some conceivable need someone will find a way to fill that need. Examples might include: an app that reads labels and advises you to buy or avoid certain products, based on your prior inputs concerning your goals (vegan, vegetarian, etc.), special dietary needs (allergies, acid reflux, etc.), and preferences (e.g. no carrageenan). And if you cannot pronounce words like carrageenan, use Google online aids such as the one at the link in endnote 237 in the References[237].

When preparing a shopping list that includes ingredients for recipes found online (see e.g. the one at the link in endnote 238 in the References)[238], in magazines, and in books be sure to read the recipes with a critical eye because many of them call for ingredients that are really not necessary (e.g. sea salt), too expensive (e.g. pine nuts), or not available (e.g. Ceylon cinnamon) at your grocery stores. And recipes frequently suggest methods of preparation that require the purchase of appliances that you may not possess (e.g. powerful high speed blender or food processor).

Recipes can have what you may consider undesirable time and temperature specifications (e.g. baking instead of microwaving sweet potatoes), and many recipes don't produce tasty results. Eventually, if you are patient and don't discard them, you might modify and improve those recipes each time you use them. To document and preserve your improvisations, consider storing the latest versions in protective plastic sleeves.

A dry erase refrigerator magnet notepad can be useful to maintain your supplies of the numerous vegetables, fruits, salad dressings, dry, frozen, and canned food, cereals and grains, spices and herbs, condiments, food wrappers, etc. However, for some readers might prefer to store the list on a cell phone or computer.

You may need cutting boards, a mandolin slicer, mezzaluna, and sharp knives to prepare salad ingredients. Choose cutting boards that are easy to keep clean and try not to dull sharp knives. Consider purchasing a salad knife, and a salad spinner.

Most readers are familiar with the essential kitchen appliances like food processors that are widely available at stores and online and there are many competitive products to choose from. Additionally, there are many less familiar useful tools and devices that you may want to check out. They are too numerous to mention. A few examples are discussed below.

To control what you eat away from home, consider purchasing a personal portable "oven" – a insulated tote that contains an electric heating pad – with approximately 150 cubic inches or about 2500 cc capacity for use in the office, job site, campsite or wherever there is an outlet. These mobile mini-ovens allow you to enjoy fresh-cooked hot meals, reheated meals or cooked prepackaged meals away from home.

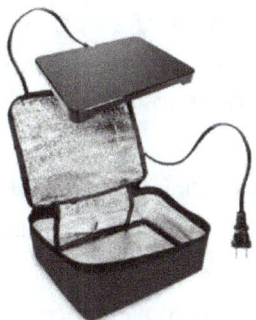

HotLogic Mini Personal Portable Oven

Another clever device is Joseph Joseph's Uni-tool. It has five functions in one tool – a slotted spoon, a turner, a solid spoon, a spatula and a cutting tool. It's made from tough nylon and is heat resistant up to 240 degrees C / 480 degrees F. It is dishwasher safe and useful for non-stick cookware.

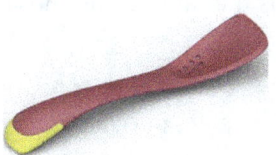

Joseph Joseph's Uni-tool

A mandolin slicer can be a very helpful time saver. Be sure to look for safety features like slip-resistant rubber feet. And an ambidextrous food safety holder that requires little pressure to hold the food in place with prongs that guard your hands from the blades.

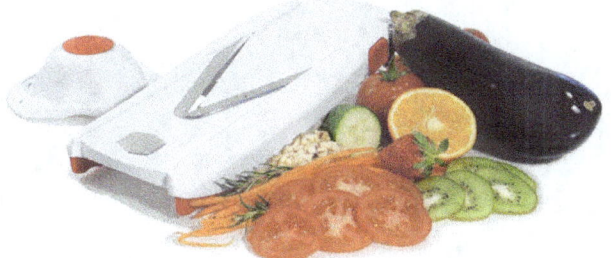

Swissmar Borner V Power Mandoline

This model provides 10 different cuts. It features a patented push button that allows size and thickness adjustment without removing the insert. But be prepared to have to trade-off the convenience of being able to clean it in a dishwasher for the performance of sharp surgical grade stainless steel blades.

Subscribe to Meal Kit Delivery Services

An alternative to cooking plant based meals at home is offered by meal kit delivery services that deliver fresh ingredients to your door, saving you time spent on meal planning and grocery shopping.

Nationwide delivery meal subscription services are offered by Blue Apron[239]. Hello Fresh[240], and Plated[241], delivering meals that are prepared and ready to be cooked at home. Hello Fresh does not offer vegan options but does deliver vegetarian meals. The Purple Carrot[242], ships vegan meals to 25 states.

Blue Apron's recipe cards include a link to an online tips page where you can find helpful how-to videos for their specific recipe from Blue Apron chefs. Plated's offers include desserts.

These services capitalize on growing demand for convenience and interest in cooking at home. They can make it easy for you to cook creative, flavorful, and satisfying vegan or vegetarian dishes.

Hire a Chef

If you don't want to invest time shopping, cooking, and acquiring the skills to prepare delicious healthful meals, consider hiring a private chef or a personal chef. A private chef is employed by one individual or family full time, and often lives-in, preparing up to three meals per day. A personal chef serves several clients, usually one per day, and provides multiple meals that are custom-designed for the client's particular requests and requirements.

Personal chefs design and execute menus for clients. They plan, purchase and prepare meals (usually once a week) either at the clients' home or in a rented professional kitchen. Meals are packaged and stored, either in the clients' refrigerator or freezer with heating-instruction labels.

According to the American Personal & Private Chef Association the current number of personal chefs is estimated at 9,000 serving 72,000 customers. And industry observers predict the number will double in the next 5 years. The typical client mix includes two-income couples with or without children, career-focused individuals, those with special dietary or health needs, seniors and those who enjoy fine dining[243].

Chapter Seven: Filling Your Shopping Cart and Stocking Your Pantry

I pushed my cart in the produce isles,
Passing colorful fruits and vegetable piles,
Neat, vibrant, fresh displays
Of spinach and kale high in vitamin K,
Fresh looking caps on shiny purple eggplants,
Life imitating art like a still life by Rembrandt,
The stoplight bell peppers made me pause for awhile,
Red, yellow, and green stacked single file,
Caramel peanut coated apples were not on my list,
But with chocolate chips too they were hard to resist.

Having a well stocked refrigerator, freezer, and pantry is essential for preparing healthful meals. Food pyramids can be useful devices to help construct shopping lists for staples to store in your refrigerator, freezer, and pantry. This concept is illustrated in this chapter with an example using the Toothsome Triangle, introduced in Chapter Four, to formulate a hypothetical shopping list. Some grocery shopping tips and suggestions are also included.

As mentioned in Chapter Two, we don't yet have readily available devices with linear programming models to optimize meals and diet options for all contingencies, including exceptions for your favorite foods or flavors. However, once you are familiar with the nutrient densities of the foods that you eat, and with their locations on the food pyramid that you use, you can rely on your brain to perform reasonable approximations without having to do the arithmetic. Your brain holds knowledge of some things that your mind cannot explicitly access. Steering your car into a parking space while talking on your cell phone is an examples of this. You execute these actions easily but without knowing the details of how you do it. For example, here is the mathematical equivalent of a calculation that your brain performs implicitly when you parallel park a car[244]:

$$\sqrt{(r^2 - l^2) + (l + k)^2 - \left(\sqrt{(r^2 - l^2) - w}\right)^2} - l - k$$

where r is the car's curb-to-curb turning circle, l is the car's wheel-base, k is the distance from the center of the front wheel to the front of the car, and w is the width of one of the parked cars, viz., the one near the front of your car once you've parked.

In addition to checking the nutrient density scores, you should occasionally determine if your meals are meeting the recommended daily values (intakes) for minerals, vitamins, and essential fats. Try to include in your daily meals the required amounts of vitamins, minerals, and omega-3 fatty acids, so you don't have to take supplements.

In the example below, we have included nutrient density values using ANDI scores that were readily available on the Internet (some scores found on the Internet may differ depending on when or where they were posted). Other nutrient density scores would also have served the purpose. The reader is encouraged to become familiar with the nutrient density scores for their foods, but it is not necessary or frequently not convenient to tag each item on a shopping list with its nutrient density score.

The following example illustrates how to populate your shopping list utilizing a food pyramid (the Toothsome Triangle) and nutrient density values together to select the ingredients listed in recipes, which can be found on the Internet, in magazines and books, and from various other sources.

Proceeding from the bottom up in the Toothsome Triangle example below:

Water Level

Recall that water occupied the bottom of the figure below the Toothsome Triangle. Water is included in many food pyramids to emphasize its role as an essential nutrient and to promote body hydration. There may be sensible reasons to purchase bottled water. Common examples include the poor water quality, the contamination of available drinking water, or the absence of convenient drinking fountains. And there are special circumstances such as drinking alkaline water to denature the pepsin in the throats of people suffering from acid reflux. Bottled water is always a better choice than diet soda or sugary drinks, which increase the risk of type 2 diabetes, heart disease, and other chronic conditions[245]. Whenever possible avoid water with added sweeteners and sugar substitutes[246]. Tap water is the first and best choice. If you want to add flavor infuse water with your favorite fruit. In the text box below we offer some cautionary advice in the event bottled water is on your shopping list.

If you can and preserve foods be aware that water is an important ingredient in successful food preservation. Hard water contains larger amounts of minerals than soft water. A certain amount of calcium and magnesium salts is desirable to set the pectins in fruits and vegetables such as in canning peaches and pears. However, large amounts of minerals can toughen peas, beans and shrivel pickles. Hard water can cause cloudy liquid in canned fruits and vegetables as the high temperatures cause the minerals to settle out of the liquid, but it is not harmful[247].

Be sure to guard against tainted food that can cause food-borne illness. Carefully inspect products and wash produce before you use it. There are new federal rules, which cover both farmers who grow fresh produce, and food importers, that are intended to prevent food-borne bacterial illness from vegetables that are often consumed raw.

The FDA is mandated under the FDA Food Safety Modernization Act to establish science-based, minimum standards for the safe growing, harvesting, packing, and holding of produce on farms to minimize contamination that could cause serious adverse health consequences or death[248].

Water

If you are concerned about the quality of your well water follow EPA's guidance: Consider testing your well for pesticides, organic chemicals, and heavy metals before you use it for the first time. Test private drinking water supplies annually for nitrate and coliform bacteria to detect contamination problems early. Test them more frequently if you suspect a problem. Be aware of activities in your watershed that may affect the water quality of your well, especially if you live in an unsewered area.

Municipal water users can contact their local water utility to get a report on water quality and call the EPA's toll-free Safe Drinking Water Hotline at 800-426-4791 or visit their website[249]. Most water utilities meet the EPA's tap water regulations, but there are many unregulated contaminants in tap water. Individual states may require additional testing.

Bottled water may not be safer than municipal supplies or furnished from a higher quality source because some vendors simple bottle tap water and the water can also be contaminated during the bottling process. The FDA sets standards for bottled water only if the water is bottled in one state and sold in another. The FDA standards regulate microbiological, physical, radiological, and chemical characteristics of the water. When the EPA promulgates a standard for a chemical or microbial contaminant for public water, the FDA must either adopt the same standard for bottled water or find that the standard is unnecessary for bottled water to maintain the safety of the water. The FDA also inspects bottled water plants and collects and analyzes samples of bottled water.

Bottled water may have to comply with the bottled water regulations of individual states, meet the state licensing requirements, and pass facilities and records inspections. Some states may test water samples and check bottled water labels for misbranding[250].

Bottling water has created significant energy and environmental concerns, and it is a very expensive alternative to tap water. If you are going to buy bottled water take the time to determine the source (e.g. municipal supply, springs, wells, surface waters), the method used to filter it (e.g. carbon, ion exchange, reverse osmosis), and the kind of plastic used to bottle it (e.g. PET or PETE, HDPE, LDPE, PVC, styrene, polypropylene)[251].

Alternatively, if you decide to filter your water, chose the kind of filter system (e.g. carbon, reverse osmosis, etc.) that has the capability to addresses your specific requirements[252]. Look for filters approved by organizations such as NSF International, UL, or the Water Quality Association and clean them in accordance with the recommendations of the manufacturer.

The agency recently finalized the first of five new federal standards that will establish the foundation of, and central framework for, the modern food safety system envisioned by Congress in the FDA Food Safety

Modernization Act[253]. You can learn more about the new rules and follow the promulgation of the remaining rules by visiting the FDA websites.

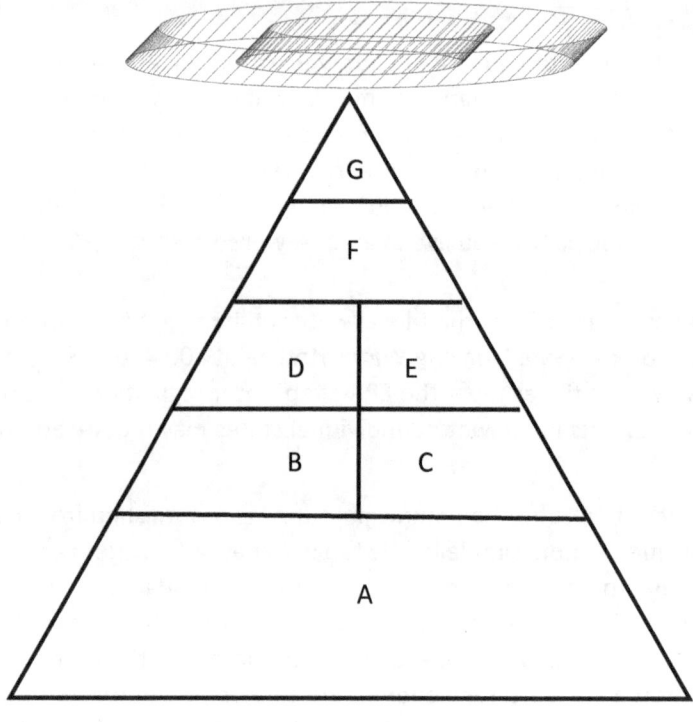

Toothsome Triangle

Plan to purchase produce that is not bruised or damaged. Store perishable fresh fruits and vegetables (like strawberries, lettuce, herbs, and mushrooms) in a clean refrigerator at a temperature of 40° F or below. And refrigerate all produce that is purchased pre-cut or peeled.

Vegetables at Base Level (A)

Watercress, arugula, kale, spinach, are just four the nutrient dense greens chosen for this shopping list. A quick search on the Internet reveals their ANDI scores are 1000, 604, 1000, and 707 respectively. Their availability can depend on which stores are visited, where the stores are located, the season, or even the day of the visit, and possibly other factors. To ensure successful shopping, we would add to the grocery list additional nutrient rich vegetables to serve as substitutes such as, collard greens, Swiss chard, green leaf lettuce, and baby bok choy. The four first choices and their substitutes can be switched with subsequent shopping trips, or exchanged with still other green vegetables, depending on your tastes.

It is desirable to have a large variety of greens but avoid purchasing more than you can use in a couple of days or more than can be frozen and stored. Fresh produce is preferred to frozen products but some perishable food will begin to decompose within a few days. If you purchased more than you can handle – e.g., a huge bag of spinach – cook it and refrigerate or freeze it.

Fruits and vegetables tend to make more ethylene as they ripen, but refrigeration helps slow the production of ethylene. Use the table of the ethylene production and sensitivity of perishable fruits and vegetables (provided in the Appendix) and separate the sensitive produce from the ethylene producers to make your produce last longer. Also, try to eat the ripest fruit first, and refrigerate produce once it is ripe.

Carefully inspect bagged and frozen products for their expiration dates. For vegetables and other produce, make note of their freshness, prices and availability at various stores in your shopping area. Try to determine when your grocer re-stocks the shelves with fresh fruits and vegetables before they begin to decompose – many grocers leave the older, picked-over produce on display up to or past the expiration dates to avoid discarding it. These considerations also apply to the other food products discussed below.

Carrots (458), mushrooms (238), red onions (109), yellow-, orange-, and red- bell peppers (265), fennel bulb (60), eggplant (149), corn (45), and cucumbers (87) complete the base level of the pyramid. Fresh vegetables are preferred but frozen, cut vegetables can serve as convenient alternatives. Yellow and orange bell peppers are frequently more expensive than red bell peppers. Fennel bulbs and packages of frozen, sliced, cleaned mushrooms can sometimes be difficult to find.

Mushrooms are not plants, they are fungi. Store mushrooms unwashed in a paper bag or paper towel in the refrigerator. Mushrooms should be cleaned and cooked before eating them because they are often grown in sterilized manure and can contain agaritine, a potential carcinogen.

Berries, Fruits and Beans (legumes) Level (B,C)

Proceeding left to right on the next level: Cranberries (34), blueberries (132), grapes (119), pomegranate (119), strawberries (182), blackberries (178), oranges (98), watermelon (91), and olives (25). Dried Cranberries and olives are readily available year-around. You can freeze berries you buy in the summer to store for the winter months. Fresh pomegranates seem to disappear from stores in spring and summer. The quality and prices of fresh berries can vary substantially among stores. You may be surprised to learn that olives are actually fruits (of olive trees).

Edamame (98), lentils (72), garbanzo (57), pinto-(61), adzuki-(84), kidney-(64), and black beans (83), are available in dry, canned, and frozen forms. Adzuki beans might be more difficult to find. Many other beans are acceptable alternatives (e.g. great northern beans (77), lima beans (69)). Edamame is a young soybean that has been harvested before the beans have had a chance to harden.

Seeds, Nuts, Grains, Cereals (D,E)

Avocado (28), walnuts (30), almonds (28), pecans (41), cashews (27), flax-(103), sunflower-(64), chia-(68), and pumpkin-(52) seeds. Selecting avocados can depend upon a number of factors including ripeness, flavor, the peeling and ripening characteristics, and oil content. Seeds and nuts are frequently available from bulk food dispensing stations but packaged products might be preferable to ensure freshness. Note that avocados are actually fleshy fruits and nuts are dry fruits.

Steel cut-, rolled- oats (54), quinoa (21), whole wheat flour (31), brown rice (28), and wheat berries (25). These are also available packaged or dispensed in bulk form, and their flavors can vary substantially among the large variety of products. The prices for Irish steel-cut oats can be twice as high in supermarket chains compared to specialty markets.

Protein, Non-Dairy and Fats Level (F)

Cholesterol free eggs (30), salmon (34), almond milk (19), cashew milk, soy milk (33), and no oil dressings. Salmon is available in fresh, frozen, canned and packaged forms. Wild and farmed raised salmon vary substantially in price, quality, and the environmental impacts of production. Price and taste will also vary among king or Chinook, sockeye, coho, pink, and Atlantic.

Federal regulators recently approved a genetically engineered salmon as fit for consumption. An Atlantic salmon has been genetically modified so that it grows to market size faster than a non-engineered farmed salmon, in as little as half the time. The salmon are not yet available for sale.

Finding and selecting no-oil dressings can be an experience that will test your skills at critically reading labels and challenge your resolve. Acceptable products without unacceptable additives are not generally found in supermarket chain stores and they can be very expensive, especially if purchased online. Flavored vinegars are fine if you don't have to avoid acidic food. If you can't find reasonably priced no-oil dressings at specialty grocers, you can try to create your own from recipes found online, in magazines, and books. Other healthful alternatives include creating salad dressing using avocado (contains oil), and hummus (contains tahini composed of olive oil and sesame paste).

Processed Plant Based Substitutes Level (G)

Also on this level are Tofu (82), tempeh (26), and seitan products, the so-called vegetarian proteins.

3 oz. servings	Tofu	Tempeh	Seitan
Protein (g)	8	16.6	18

Here you are faced with make versus buy decisions. If you haven't tasted them and didn't enjoy or didn't want to try restaurant dishes containing these products you might get past the psychological hurdles and become more comfortable with the idea of eating them if you try making them from scratch. Some things seem to taste better when you make them yourself, because psychologically you've seen everything that goes into making it, so you appreciate it more. However, be advised that there is a learning curve and first attempts usually do not meet expectations, but keep trying until you discover what went wrong or how to make tasty versions.

Another strategy is to delay purchasing the ingredients needed to make your own batches until you find out how tofu, tempeh, and seitan are supposed to taste by buying the commercial packaged versions for your immediate use in recipes found online, in magazines, or books. However, the taste of the commercial products can also vary considerably, so it pays to persevere and try several different products. Similarly, you can sample tofu, tempeh, and seitan at buffets but keep in mind that restaurant food can vary also from horrible to delicious. Often the presence or absence or too little or too much of just one spice or herb can be the determining factor.

Typical Process for Making Tofu

Soak dried soybeans in water for about 8 hours (or overnight). After soaking, grind the soybeans with their soaking water in a food processor, until the beans are ground fine.

Add the ground soybeans to boiling water. Reduce to medium heat, and keep the mixture almost at a boil, stirring continuously, until a layer of foam forms on top.

Strain the bean mixture through cheesecloth-lined colander and reserve the liquid (soy milk). Gather up the sides of the cheesecloth and twist it closed to squeeze out as much liquid as possible. Discard cheesecloth and solids.

Dissolve a coagulant (e.g. nigari (magnesium chloride), gypsum (calcium sulfate), epsom salts (magnesium sulfate)) in water.

Cook the soy milk over low heat, stirring continuously until the temperature of the soy milk is between 150 and 155 degrees, then add half of the coagulant mixture to the soy milk, stirring vigorously before adding the remaining coagulant mixture and stirring gently. When the soy milk starts to coagulate, cover the mixture and let it sit for about 15 minutes.

Transfer the coagulated soy milk into a cloth-lined colander (or tofu press or loaf pan). Fold the cloth over the top of the coagulated soy milk, and place a plate on it and then add a weight on top. Let the tofu stand for about 15 minutes to press out any excess water.

Place it in a refrigerator to chill and firm slightly, about an hour. Serve it or store it in fresh, cold water in the refrigerator for up to three days.

Typical Process for Making Tempeh

Place the soy beans in a bowl and cover them with water and optionally add a small amount of vinegar. Then soak them overnight.

De-husk the soy beans and remove the skins the following day.
Cook the beans in water (optionally with some vinegar) then drain the water.
On the next dry the beans and allow them to cool.

To inoculate the beans with a starter culture that contains Rhizopus mold spores, add the starter to the cooled, dry beans and mix it well. Then place the inoculate beans in perforated zip-top bags and incubate the bags at 85°- 90°F for 24 to 48 hours.

The tempeh is ready to be refrigerated when the inside of the bags are white and solid. The beans will have become a single mass held together by the white spores.

Refrigerating the tempeh stops the fermentation. The soybean tempeh can be made with the addition of seed such as sesame, flax, or sunflower.

Typical Process for Making Seitan

Combine vital wheat gluten, granulated garlic, and ground ginger and mix thoroughly.

Combine water or vegetable broth, reduced sodium tamari, and toasted sesame oil (optional) and add to the dry mixture.

Mix with a fork until the dough reaches a kneadable consistency. Knead a couple of dozen times, and then let the dough rest 3-5 minutes. Next, wet your hands (to prevent gluten from sticking) and knead another dozen times. Let the dough rest while preparing the broth.

Combine water, reduced-sodium tamari, and ginger (optional) in a large pot with a lid. Bring broth to a boil, add gluten dough pieces, and reduce to a simmer and cover. Check occasionally and add more water if needed.

Wet your hands and a knife; cut gluten into 6-8 pieces and pull into thin strips. Simmer the gluten in broth for 45-60 minutes.

Note that the flavor of the broth will determine the flavor of the seitan. The addition of herbs such as herbes de Provence is highly recommended.

Convenience food versions of meat and fish substitutes can vary considerably in quality and taste. Carefully read the labels. If the ingredients are acceptable purchase the smallest package that is available and follow the instructions for preparation. Some might pass your taste tests. You might have to add to or mask the flavor of bland products with vegetable, spices, sauces, or substitute cheese products.

At this level of the pyramid it is important to keep in mind the need to limit or try to avoid processed fats and added sugars. Regardless of their sources, all oils are processed food that have lost their fiber and nutrients. Notwithstanding that olive oil is rich in monounsaturated fat and the relatively good sources of healthy unsaturated fats like, soy, corn, sunflower, and peanut oil, they all provide 120 calories per tablespoon of empty calories. Added sugars are also nutrient deficient substances that are rapidly absorbed into the bloodstream.

Spices and Herbs Halo

Basil (518), bay leaves, Ceylon cinnamon, lavender, cilantro (481), lemon grass (55), oregano (426), parsley (381), rosemary (84), and thyme (422). These and many other healthful spices can ensure that your successful journey to healthful eating will be toothsome and delicious. Some spices and herbs can be grown at home. Except perhaps for Ceylon cinnamon, they are readily available in the spices sections of grocery stores. Fresh varieties of basil, cilantro, parsley, etc., can be found in the produce sections. Look for fresh aroma and bright green leaves and avoid damaged, dried out, and browning leaves. Try not to purchase more than you can use before they begin to decompose.

Dried packaged products have long shelf lives, but to preserve their strength avoid purchasing more supplies than needed for a year. Keep in mind that you will be visiting grocery stores frequently through the year, so there will be many opportunities to restock your supplies. And obviously there is no need to discard any items simply because they are over a year old. Plan to store your spices and seasoning blends in air tight containers, preferably in a cool dark place. To protect them from heat and moisture; do not store them above your stove or dishwasher. Avoid exposure to steaming food by dispensing small quantities from your hand or a ramekin. The quality and prices of dried, packaged products and bulk dispensers can vary considerably. Good values may be found online.

Note that the Toothsome Triangle example was not meant to generate a comprehensive grocery shopping list. Many more items may be included depending on what is already available in your kitchen and your past culinary experiences. Garlic and olive oil are obvious examples. Consider substituting whole grain flat bread wraps for bread, and perhaps diary-free cheese products and plant-based products that mimic the taste of chicken, beef, or pork. Note also that some items, particularly the diary-free cheese products, can spoil quickly in the refrigerator after the packages are opened.

As you examine appealing recipes to prepare shopping lists try to include contingencies for substituting (indicated by the symbol **s**) for ingredients such as jicama (s water chestnuts), currants (s raisins), saffron (s turmeric), or pine nuts (s walnuts), that might not be available, or too expensive, or are not acceptable. Lists of ingredient substitutions are available on the Internet[254].

More Shopping Tips

We would be remiss not to suggest taking advantage of exceptional values that can be found at food warehouses, for items such as fresh and frozen berries, apples, raisins, brown rice, hemp seeds, sesame seeds, olives, roasted red peppers, frozen microwaveable quinoa and kale, almonds, walnuts, pecans, pistachios, pomegranates, English cucumbers, almond butter, bell peppers, mushrooms, spicy black bean veggie burgers, salmon, etc. And it pays to visit the tasting stations to sample unfamiliar products.

Build your shopping list with creative cooking in mind. The creative ways in which you prepare and combine the ingredients can be key to crafting delicious, healthful meals.

We suggest that you plan to include in your shopping list provisions for using a large assortment of ingredients in each of your meals, in addition to planning for variety among you daily meals. It is said that Aristotle coined the phrase, *"The whole is greater than the sum of its parts."* If he was thinking about food we could credit him with having described the junction where delicious meets healthful. Watercress, arugula, kale, spinach, the four nutrient dense greens chosen to illustrate the components of our shopping list can be used separately to create a tasty salad, for instance – spinach salads are popular examples.

However, we recommend chopping and mixing <u>all four of them together</u> to form the base of a big salad. Add to that base thin slices or chunks of <u>all three colored bell peppers</u>, plus dried cranberries or fresh blueberries, walnuts or other nuts, sliced English cucumber, flax seed, sesame seeds, sunflower seeds, and a flavorful dressing with herbs and spices. And add to the salad any other ingredients that you savor from any level of the pyramid and you will have created a toothsome salad.

The same multi-component concept can be applied to chilies, soups, stews, sandwiches, and breakfast meals. One that you are familiar with from the Preface includes an example of breakfast foods, viz., various combinations of steel cut oats, quinoa and flax, bananas, oranges, raisins, dates, walnuts, pecans, almonds, almond milk, cashew milk, soy milk and cinnamon.

The combinations of ingredients can create remarkably different flavors and textures. That idea is dramatically realized in the preparation of tofu, tempeh, and seitan where the clever use of spices and herbs can make something that is meant to mimic animal products become virtually indistinguishable, or taste even better than the real thing. Seitan crafted to mimic chicken can be made to taste better than chicken, but without careful preparation it can taste like a wet sponge that was used to mop spilled soup. Experiment with various spices –e.g. mixed spices can dramatically enhance Seitan Mushroom Stroganoff.

Time and Money Tradeoffs

Grocery shopping trips can easily require two or three hours, not including the time spent traveling from your home to the first store and returning to your home from the last store. Preparing large multi-ingredient breakfast meals or salads can take half an hour. Making seitan from scratch will occupy several hours. Preparing meals from various recipes frequently entails several hours and some recipes extend the process overnight or over several days. For example, tofu preparation calls for soybeans to be soaked overnight before 6-7 hours preparation the next day, and making tempeh involves soaking the soybeans overnight plus additional steps including incubation that necessitate a day or two, and sometimes longer.

However, many healthful meals can be quickly assembled in as little as five minutes. Faux chicken and cheese sandwiches with lettuce and tomato or fire roasted red peppers can be prepared in less time than it takes to go through a fast food pickup station. Add a bowl of bean soup, some carrots and an apple and you have quickly created a tasty lunch. But remember to eat it slowly, take about 20-30 minutes to allow your brain to catch up with the signals from your stomach that it is full (giving the body's intricate hormonal cross-talk system enough time to work), and possibly head-off cravings for the frozen dark chocolate truffle cashew milk or frozen mint chocolate chip almond milk in your freezer.

With the adoption of a plant based diet you can expect to spend a great deal more time shopping for groceries and your grocery bills will be significantly higher. However, the value of your meals will be much higher when you take into account the health benefits of adopting a plant based diet. And the cost of your groceries should certainly be much less than the costs of eating out. According to Zagat's 2015 Dining Trend Survey, the national average cost per person per dinner out was $39.40. In 2014, one source estimated that, *"the average American would save $36.75 per person per week by moving all of their meals from restaurants to home-prepared meals"*[255]. Another claimed in 2013 that Americans went out for lunch on average twice a week and they spent $936 annually[256].

A Review of Your Journey to Healthful Eating

This book has provided you with knowledge concerning the health benefits of plant based diets, and the health impacts of poor diet choices. You have became familiar with the molecular nature of human digestion, appetite, and energy metabolism, and the application of the nutrient density concept to profile or rate foods. You have received guidance on avoiding or limiting harmful substances in foods, food products, additives, and nutritional supplements, and learned the key attributes and nourishing characteristics of healthful foods including, for example, the relationship of fruit and vegetable consumption with wellness and the development of chronic disease.

Armed with that knowledge, you selected or created a healthful, plant based diet style that allows you to meet your personal goals. You might have tailored an existing diet style or fashioned your own healthful diet style to meet your needs and tastes. In either case you should be confident that it is a healthful, plant based diet style which you expect to faithfully follow and enjoy.

Next, you adapted for your use one or more of the published food pyramids or crafted your own food pyramid, augmented with published values for the nutrient density of selected foods to formulate a shopping list for staples to store in your refrigerator, freezer, and pantry, and for use in planning meals. Using that information and knowledge you are ready to prepare and enjoy you own healthful, plant based meals or select healthful prepared meals at restaurants or from other sources. A roadmap for your journey is illustrated below.

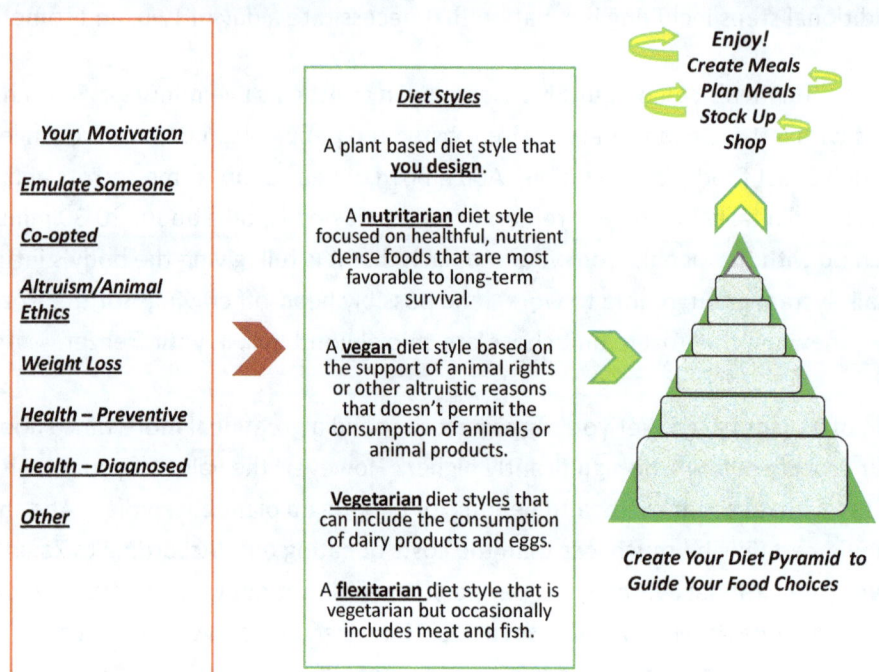

Chapter Eight:

Dining at Restaurants & Dining with Friends and Relatives

It can be rewarding to experience plant based foods prepared in many different ways. Plant-based food options are traditionally available in some ethnic restaurants including: Chinese restaurants that serve vegetable and tofu-based dishes. And plant-based dishes appear on Thai, Vietnamese, Middle-Eastern, and Indian restaurant menus. Even traditional American restaurants are attempting to respond to the growing demand for healthful options. But the food quality and number of menu offerings can vary considerably. Hence, you might have to ask the restaurant staff to accommodate your special needs. We recently heard someone placing an order ask for *"beef with vegetables in black bean sauce and hold the beef."*

Prior planning is prudent to avoid unpleasant experiences. Make sure the business still exist and check on the safety of the restaurant's location. A trial run may help answer concerns about traffic, parking, security and other potential issues. Restaurant guides, reviews in newspapers and magazines, and patron's online reviews can be very helpful, particularly reviews of the same restaurant from several independent sources. But because we all have different tastes even the most glowing endorsements by plant-based food advocates will not guarantee meeting or exceeding your expectations.

With or without information from reviews carefully examine the restaurant's menu online or at the restaurant before eating there. When you call for reservations don't hesitate to ask questions about the menu offerings, how the food is prepared and the ingredients – particularly if you are vegan. Look for foods prepared by baking, broiling, braising, grilling or other ways that don't add extra fat. Find out if any of the items that you are considering are prepared with butter, trans-fat margarine, dairy, fish, meat, eggs, or cheese. If you don't see references to healthy fats, condiments, or dairy substitutes that interest you on the menu, like avocado, hummus, or soy milk, ask if they are available. Can you get a larger portion of vegetables and a smaller portion of the main dish? Ask if they will accommodate substitutions or a special meal order. Chefs may be better prepared to entertain a special order if they are asked a day or so in advance of your visit. Also look for nutrition information about the menu items.

Be aware that restaurant reviews posted on the Internet, and web pages that include attractive menus can frequently mask a dive with poor accommodations, bad service, and unpalatable food. It may not be a good idea to rely exclusively on a review article. Restaurant reviews can be like movie reviews, you can't always depend on them to be accurate and helpful. So, unless they are telling you that roaches are crawling on the tables and up the walls, the Health Department has shut the place down, or that you are likely to be mugged at that location, take the review with a grain of salt. Even the information about nearby parking can be totally wrong.

We visited a restaurant that frequently received rave reviews in one of America's leading daily newspapers, for its vegan sandwiches and bakery products, but the reviewer cautioned that nearby parking was not available during weekday lunch hours. It turned out that there was abundant parking just across the street in a huge, multi-level parking garage, albeit with poor lighting and dank surroundings that gave cause for concern about safety. The restaurant is a dive. The display case for what was supposed to be prized bakery products was nearly empty, with just one stale looking cupcake. The service was almost non-existent. Just one other customer was seated at a table with a finished plate that had not been cleared. We waited twenty five minutes for what the reviewer touted as the restaurant's best sandwich to arrive. After several bites of the sandwich we discovered a broken toothpick buried in the middle of the unremarkable bean burger.

Many restaurants have thoughtfully responded to the needs of vegetarians, with vegetarian menu options. However, other use the adjective "veggie" loosely to offer deceptively unhealthy choices. Don't be fooled by tasty veggie burgers that contain more calories than cheese burgers or grilled chicken burgers and are not healthful. The patties can be held together with oil or lard, deep fried, slathered in creamy sauces, and topped with mushrooms saturated with butter or oil and various kinds of cheese. The buns can be coated with oil or butter before they are grilled or fried.

Order plant based menu items that are consistent with your new diet strategy. The menus may vary from familiar menu options that are completely in line with meals you have tasted elsewhere or prepared at home, to dishes that you have never heard of that contain ingredients you have never tasted. New gustatory experiences can be highly rewarding, successful adventures where you enjoy delicious, healthful meals, and learn about exciting new foods that you can prepare at home, or they might be disappointing.

Your strategy for eating at traditional American restaurants should focus on avoiding unhealthful foods and trying to build a tasty meal from the selection of available options. For example, start by asking for water and avoid free bread, rolls, biscuits, or any chips and dips, but try to substitute carrots, celery, or other vegetables that are available. Bean soup, pea soup, or vegetable based soups or side salads might be acceptable as starters if they don't have excessive salt. And you might select a healthful side salad with a vinaigrette dressing, which should be furnished separately in a small container. However, it is better to start with a large salad that has a variety of vegetables, fruits, nuts, seeds, olives, and grains and no-oil dressing. Flavored vinegar with a small amount of olive oil are ok. And possibly add salmon. Remember to eat the meal slowly.

The following illustrates a hypothetical example of making the best of a bad situation at a popular chain restaurant. This might have occurred if you happened to dine at the restaurant that won the 2015 Xtreme Eating Awards, an annual contest by the Center for Science in the Public Interest designed to highlight the chain restaurant menu items with the highest calorie, saturated and trans fat, sodium, and added sugar counts. The award winning meal contained a total of 3,600 calories, which included an 890 calorie margarita and a combination of coconut shrimp, shrimp and shrimp linguine alfredo with a Caesar salad, French fries and a biscuit that added 2,710 calories and 6,530 mg of sodium.

Suppose you unexpectedly had to eat lunch at that famous restaurant. Could you choose a menu item that does not *"exemplify the kind of gargantuan restaurant meal that promotes obesity, diabetes and other diet-related diseases"* – borrowing the characterization of the award winning combination? The characteristics the Classic Caesar Salad is shown in the table below.

Classic Caesar Salad		Daily Values	%DV
Calories	540	2000	27
Total Fat (g)	50	65	77
Sat. Fat (g)	9	20	45
Trans. Fat (g)	0	0	
Cholesterol (mg)	40	300	13
Sodium (mg)	1140	2400	47.5
Carb (g)	15	300	5
Fiber (g)	5	25	20
Protein (g)	8	50	16

This menu item, which also contains 2 grams of sugar, is survivable and you might be able to make it a lot more nutritious by asking your server to add and delete ingredients to tailor the salad to your requirements. It is a better option that just giving up and choosing something far worse.

If the big salad is not your main dish or you must order additional food, look for vegetarian or vegan menu items that are becoming available in traditional restaurants. Otherwise, ask for extra vegetables on the house salad and select salmon for a main course, with one or more vegetable sides. Or just combine enough vegetable side dishes to form the meal. Also select fresh fruits for dessert (or appetizer). Finally, if you have just begun the transition to a plant-based diet it may be a good idea to avoid eating at traditional restaurants to minimize the risk of disappointment and frustration and the temptation of unhealthful comfort food.

It is reasonable to expect authentic vegan restaurants to be the places where you can enjoy delicious, healthful meals, learn about exciting new foods and discover how to prepare them at home. However, dining at vegan restaurants also requires careful planning, particularly regarding their locations and menu pricing. Don't assume the menu options or quality of the food are typical of vegan dining or even consistent at the same restaurant. You can expect the ingredients and preparation to be safe and healthful but be aware of the calorie content of the drinks and desserts.

Some vegan restaurants are collocated with specialty grocery stores that have excellent produce, packaged, bulk and frozen food, and even salad bars and buffets. You can frequently learn the ingredients of the buffet items from the labels, but few businesses will provide recipes for their buffet items. Buffet establishments and salad bars can offer delicious meals particularly in cities catering to large lunch time clients. But buffets do present some special health risk challenges including hot and cold foods not maintained at proper temperatures, improper bare hand contact with food by clientele, inadequate personal cleanliness, flies, evidence of roaches, and customers handle the same serving utensils[257].

Salad bars in supermarkets and specialty grocery stores also can be good places to explore the tastes of unfamiliar food, but the quality of some of the food can be very low because of age, mishandling or contamination. Look for signs of freshness (just made) and watch for potential sources of contamination.

Various local public health departments regularly inspect businesses serving food to ensure restaurants and other food retail outlets are following safe food handling procedures. Many do not. Some links to local inspectors can be found in the References at endnote number 258[258].

Finally, it may be helpful and possibly enjoyable to sample the vegan menu options at chain restaurants such as Chop't, Freshii, Zoës Kitchen, Veggie Grill, Native Foods Café, Lyfe Kitchen, Sweetgreen, and possibly others[259]. And there are well known independent vegetarian[260], and vegan restaurants, like Vedge[261], located in cities throughout the world. Also, look for vegan food trucks, such as the prize-winning Cinnamon Snail food truck[262,263].

Dining with Friends or Relatives

Jamie, a tea connoisseur, who suffers from acid reflex is not supposed to drink coffee or tea but she is allowed to drink chamomile *"tea,"* an herbal infusion. Jamie carries with her chamomile tea bags, which she uses to brew tea when visiting friends. She also takes chamomile tea bags to restaurants where they are pleased to provide her with a cup of hot water for her tea. Jamie's clever strategy can adapted for use by any of us for occasions when we are dining with friends or relatives and our hosts aren't known to normally consume, prepare, or serve plant based meals.

Dining with friends or relatives who don't normally consume, prepare, or serve plant based meals might require some skillful planning, coordinating, and preparation, but with successful execution you and your hosts can share many rewarding experiences.

The following are some time-tested suggestions: Ask your host whether there are particular dishes you might bring to complement the menu. And let your host know what food you are planning to bring. Be sure that any cooking and storage arrangements are easily accommodated, not awkward, or unwelcomed. The key is to prepare something easily portable that requires minimal assembling at the other end. For example, are there going to be adequate provisions for storing fruit/vegetable trays, large salad bowls, large baking dishes or baking casseroles? Make sure your activities do not generate strong cooking aromas from sulfur-rich vegetables like garlic, onions, cabbage, broccoli, Brussels sprouts and asparagus.

If you bring extra food to share leave it to the host to suggest that others may try some of the food that you are eating. Stick with dishes you have perfected. Don't use this venue to experiment with new or difficult recipes because you might not be able to recover from embarrassing mistakes.

Try to keep things low-key and avoid calling attention to your special needs. You don't have to be apologetic. Strive to feel comfortable with what you are eating but not uncomfortable or judgmental about what other people are eating. Do not attempt to proselytize your host and other guests. Refrain from discussing your dietary preferences unless the conversation is initiated by the host. Aim for light-hearted conversations. Try to recognize the difference between questions prompted by genuine curiosity and small talk. Keep your responses brief but genuine and cheerfully segue from personal questions to other topics. And, as always, try to avoid becoming engaged in flat, boring inappropriate personal conversations that will spoil your appetite.

Since everyone has different tastes, different friends and different relatives, we will refrain from suggesting recipes for occasions when you are dining with friends or relatives and your hosts aren't known to normally consume, prepare, or serve plant based meals. Instead, we are providing a few examples of food to take to the gathering that might help to stimulate your thoughts.

Breakfast or Brunch:

If you want to avoid dairy products, consider taking your own tea bags, almond milk, cashew milk, or soy milk – which are available in single serving size, aseptic containers.

Single serving pouches of oatmeal are available at grocery stores, including several flavored varieties. There are even individual pouches containing steel cut oatmeal with flax. All you need is boiling water. But you can also take along some nuts, seeds, raisins, dried cranberries, an apple, banana, or other fruit to add to the oatmeal. And remember to include spices such as Ceylon cinnamon.

Another obvious breakfast alternative is to prepare a fruit cup, or a fruit tray composed of fresh cut fruits.

The variety of breakfast sandwiches is limited only by your imagination. Try sandwich size whole grain flat breads instead of bread or rolls. Or, whole grain bagels.

Fill the sandwich with your favorite combinations of vegan cream cheese, slices or spread, and bacon substitute, plant based burger style patties, roasted red pepper, chickpeas, almond butter, etc.

Prepare salads with wheat berries, or farro and add blueberry, nuts, and seeds. Or create a farro bowl with quinoa, arugula, roasted sweet potatoes, mushrooms, and pumpkin seeds. And you can add tofu to salads or wraps.

Lunch or Dinner:

Popular lunches include sandwiches, soup, salad, plus fruit and combinations thereof. Again, you might prefer sandwich size whole grain flat breads instead of bread or rolls, to budget calories for other items. Or if you are planning to share your meal you can create wraps. Prepared wraps are frequently available in grocery stores and delis, but you might have to order them tailored to your dietary requirements.

Consider selecting options from among the examples presented in Chapter Five of plant-based meals that contain all of the essential amino acids: brown rice and beans; peanut butter and whole wheat bread; cornbread and pinto beans; refried beans with wheat or corn tortillas; and falafel and whole wheat pita.

There are several different plant based, burger style chicken and beef substitute products available in the refrigerated and frozen foods sections of grocery stores. They are easy to prepare and some can be microwaved in as little as 90 seconds. Garnish them with roasted red pepper, guacamole, romaine, cheese substitutes, or whatever interests you.

Multi-bean vegetable chilies, or vegetable soups with quinoa and kale are easy to prepare and transport. Add tofu, tempeh, or seitan chicken style strips. Garnish with cilantro, basil, or other herbs.
There are many possible variations for salads featuring wheat berry, farro, or other grains, spinach or other greens, with strawberry or other berries, and possibly with nuts and seeds. And, of course, numerous ways to create pasta salads – including whole wheat pasta or quinoa pasta.

Not only are items in a tray or casserole conveniently housed in one container, they can also be par-cooked and finished off under the grill or in the oven. Vegetable lasagna is a popular dish; consider making enough to share with everyone.

Or bring a vegetable tray, including fennel bulbs, carrots, celery, broccoli, tomatoes, a fruit tray, or hummus or guacamole dip for appetizers.

Hone your skills crafting a huge vegetable salad comprised of three or more greens (e.g. watercress, arugula, spinach), mushrooms, seeds, nuts, berries, and colorful bell peppers. And consider adding red onions, peas, or corn.

You can get many more ideas by scanning the menus of popular vegan restaurants, visiting the buffets at specialty markets, and searching online recipes using key words such as "plant-based," "vegan," or "vegetarian" diet recipes with Google hits usually exceeding one million results.

Chapter Nine: Plan Ahead and Be Prepared

"The roughest roads often lead to the top." — Christina Aguilera

Your transition to a plant based diet may not be easy. It can require spending a lot more of your time grocery shopping, planning meals, and cooking. And the conversion could call for sacrifices like giving up most, if not all, comfort foods, and halting your unhealthful eating habits. A diet style change is a major undertaking that requires commitment, patience, and perseverance.

The time and effort required for the transition can depend on many factors such as where you live and how much effort you put into planning and shopping. Unless you happen to live close to top notch restaurants and take-out delis with superb plant based food selections, the transition will not be quick and easy. It is more likely that delicious prepared vegan or vegetarian foods will not be conveniently available, and affordable.

Some excellent restaurant do have a few vegan/vegetarian selections on their menus; however, there are very few excellent vegan/vegetarian restaurants in most US cities and towns. Although we had no difficulty compiling a long list of excellent restaurants for most large US cities, it was challenging to compile a list of even three excellent vegan restaurants in most US cities.

Regardless of location, you may want to delay searching for good vegan/vegetarian restaurants and eating out until you have begun to enjoy eating big salads and have successfully crafted at least one hot healthful meal. Try to eat huge home-made salads for a week or so before going to vegan restaurants or attempting to prepare vegan sandwiches, chili, or other dishes with tempeh, soy, or seitan, so as to allow your taste preference to adapt for an appreciation of more subtle flavors.

After a few weeks of plant based dieting give some thought to planning your meals to avoid getting into a rut with boring meal routines. Consider eating out occasionally, taking breaks from your meals at home. You may discover new plant based meal alternatives by exploring new menu options at familiar restaurants and new vegan or vegetarian restaurants or food trucks. Visits to some vegan and vegetarian restaurant can provide new ideas and inspiration to create delicious meals at home.

If you want to eat healthful home cooked meal but don't have time to prepare them during the work week, make large batches of food on weekends and refrigerate or freeze portions for your weekday meals.

Be aware that the transition is a period of time when you are most likely to be caught off guard. During the course of most people's day there are many times when the choice of acceptable healthful food and beverages is very limited. You can anticipate such instances by planning in advance your daily eating activities. These may include foreseeing the need for meals or snacks at home, at work, entertainment venues (sports, theater, concerts, etc.), when traveling by car, train, plane, ship, and hiking, camping, etc.

Also carefully consider your meal plans for business or pleasure trips. Don't get stuck having to eat breakfast at a doughnut shop or meals at a hotel that has a poor selection and unhealthful foods. Avoid going to ice cream, yogurt and other dessert shops, and restaurants with menus that have no healthy food items. When you travel to distant places, allow extra time and focus more effort on choosing where and what you are going to eat at your destinations. And consider alternative options like taking along food in a personal portable oven (which may also be useful if you brown-bag lunch at work).

Seek Tasty Food

Strive to select high quality food products during your transition. You will want to avoid the unpleasant experience of eating "fake" foods like veggie hamburgers that taste like cardboard, are too soft to stay together –like a sloppy joes – and fall apart in your hands as your are trying to eat them. Or food that has a bad after taste. But endeavor not to let bad experiences thwart your transition.

Finding tasty new healthful food and avoiding distasteful products can be challenging. There are many vegan and vegetarian products available in grocery stores, and supermarkets that do not taste good, particularly frozen foods. Take advantage of the limited opportunities to sample new food items at tasting stations in big box stores and grocery stores. If you can't taste samples, buy the smallest package to avoid wastage. Try different brands of products to find the ones you like.

It helps to get guidance from someone you know with tastes similar to yours who can suggest where to get a good vegan/ vegetarian meal based on his/her experience. Just as is the case with conventional menu items, you can encounter a vegan/vegetarian restaurant meal or menu item that is not prepared correctly, not fresh, and a horrible representation of what it should be. Unfortunately, if that is your first taste it can be a turn-off experience, literally leaving a bad taste in your mouth.

Fruits and vegetables are obviously not exempt from quality and taste issues. There is in nature a great deal of variability in quality and taste, otherwise we wouldn't have idioms like sour grapes and rotten apples. One of the best times to start the transition to a plant based diet style is when high quality fresh produce is available in your shopping area.

Carefully approach your first encounter with new foods, but if the experience is disappointing, keep trying – you will discover that perseverance pays off.

Visit Your Doctor

Unless your health is already excellent, you should expect that it will improve significantly with the transition to a plant based diet. Conversely, if you have health issues that disappear after adopting a plant based diet style and you subsequently abandon healthful eating and return to your previous diet style, you can expect your old health issues to return and possibly to develop new health problems. Consider getting a physical exam. Discuss your changing eating habits with your primary care doctor and other physicians you visit so they can watch for improvements in existing conditions, identify possibly signs or symptoms of any diet related anomalies, ensure adequate intakes of certain vitamins and minerals, and change your medications or manage associated medical complications.

Work with your doctor to tailor a diet to address food allergies, acid reflux, interstitial cystitis or other conditions that require dietary restrictions. The resulting dietary restrictions on spices, nuts, salad dressings, and many other foods can hinder your progress. Creative alternatives are needed to address the restrictions.

Be prepared to shop for another doctor if your current physician does not respond appropriately. If, for example, after you report your plans for a transition to a vegan lifestyle, he/she gives you a computer generated form that advises patients to follow the Mediterranean diet, you know there has been a communications failure – perhaps the doctor was distracted, too busy, stressed, etc.

Build a Healthful Food Inventory

While several diets call for starting the transition with meals or procedures designed to "detoxify" your body, we reiterate that you must create your own menus based on your goals and tastes. Diets, fasts, or procedures that proponents claim are necessary to reset your metabolism, remove unwanted pounds, and eliminate so-called "toxins" from the body are at best unnecessary and at worst potentially harmful. There's no concrete evidence that any of these detoxing methods actually rid your body of harmful substances[264].

The cleansing should begin in your kitchen. You can empty your shelves, refrigerator, and freezer of all non-healthful foods by giving them to charitable organizations, trashing them, eating them as soon as possible or, if you don't mind delaying your transition, eating them gradually as you phase them out and restock with healthful foods.

Consider using blending and mixing to gradually increase the amounts of food you don't prefer as you change your taste preferences and learn to appreciate more subtle flavors. For example, gradually replacing milk in your meals with cashew milk, almond milk, or soy milk. Or, add brown sugar to your steel cut oatmeal and gradually phase out the brown sugar by substituting raisins, dates, walnuts, or blueberries. Or replacing the cream cheese on your bagel with vegan cream cheese, the bacon with seitan bacon, and the regular flour bagel with a whole grain bagel.

Your food inventory should reflect a strategy that includes provisions for healthy snacks and quick meal options as well as supplies for meals that require more time and labor. Examples are the various types of meat substitutes and vegan protein sources, veggie burgers, bean burgers, frozen/canned fruit and vegetables. Stock up on a variety of off the shelf low sodium vegetable soups and vegan ingredients to create soups and chilies so you are not forced to eat the readily available low nutritional, harmful foods that you are trying to avoid. Keep ample supplies of fresh fruits and vegetables that you like and try fresh fruits and vegetables that you haven't eaten before. Also include a variety of nuts and seeds. You can turn to fresh fruits, nuts, and seeds when you need a snack or as alternatives to candy and desserts.

Approach food selection constantly vigilant of the nutritional values—don't waste your appetite on empty calories and unhealthy alternatives.

Expect to spend a lot of time stocking and restocking your pantry because you will probably discover that no single grocery store will have what you need. Learn how to select the freshest produce. Focus on quality instead of price, but be sure to compare the prices different stores charge for the same items. Keep in mind that the shelf life for the produce can be less than a week, so don't purchase more perishable food than you will use. Choose produce carefully—carefully inspect big packages of fruits before buying them. Read the expiration dates on the bagged vegetables, the refrigerated products, and other perishables. Avoid buying products near or later than expiration date (some stores will leave expired products on their shelves). Avoid purchasing bagged vegetables without an expiration date. Strive to become an informed shopper by becoming familiar with the products, prices, and quality at each of the stores where you shop.

Pace the Transition

If you are overweight aim to proceed with deliberate speed. Otherwise, you can switch to a plant based diet over any timeframe or through any path you desire. As discussed in Chapter One, you might prefer to transition in a step-wise manner through any plant based diet style(s) before arriving at your destination. The rate at which you switch to a plant based diet does not have to be a reflection of your commitment or determination.

For the transition it may help to plan to choose from among alternatives that are similar to what you have been eating. For instance, if you eat cereal and milk in the mornings, you might want to eat cereal (like various oatmeals, whole grain wheat, blends, etc.) and cashew, soy or almond milk (or blends until you eliminate the animal milk). Substitute for butter vegan dairy-free spreads; for eggs—scrambled tofu. If you don't generally eat salads at lunch, start eating lunch with small salads and gradually increase the size of the salads as you diminish other items like sandwiches. Or substitute for conventional sandwiches a half of a peanut butter or almond butter sandwich on whole grain bread. And also add fruits like apples, bananas, pears, etc. Fennel bulbs, celery, carrots, and other vegetables can be tasty snacks. For dinner create the largest salad that you can eat (don't overeat salad or any other meal items) with the goal of making the salad your dinner meal. If you are still hungry after eating the salad, you can also eat other hot, room temperature, or cold meal items—in moderation, of course. Yet another alternative is to create a large meal, such as a tofu-spinach lasagna, to provide food for several people or feed you for several days. But be sure to use whole wheat lasagna, soy milk, etc.

Up for a challenge? Try going "cold turkey." In addition to avoiding the traditional comfort foods and junk foods, consider halting immediately the consumption of all foods with trans fats, saturated fats from animals, meats, dairy products, and fruit juices, and replacing them in your meals with plant based food, especially whole foods. Granted, it can be an unpleasant way to stop addictive eating habits but it is a fast way to begin to realize the rewards. And that should also help you keep focused on planning the transition to a plant based diet.

But don't overdo it. Set a pace that is reasonable and not too uncomfortable for you. As you transition to eating more high-fiber foods like fruits and vegetables, try to gradually increase the amount of daily fiber. Changing too quickly from a low-fiber diet to a very high-fiber diet can cause bloating, gas, and constipation. A more gradual transition allows the bowels and colon to adjust to the change. And it is important to drink a lot of water. Increasing your fiber without increasing water in your diet can actually cause constipation because the fiber needs water to bulk up the stool and keep it soft.

Learn from your mistakes and don't try to make excuses for falling off the wagon. If you do happen to eat something that you should not have eaten, don't give up for the day and continue to eat other food you should avoid. Try to make up for the transgression by picking up the pace of eliminating other unhealthful food from your diet, skipping a meal, or fashioning your next meals from the most nutritious foods at the lowest levels of the food pyramid. But try not to let yourself feel deprived. Recognize the difference between rationalizations and valid circumstances that delay your progress. Be patient and persistent. Don't let unanticipated events that threaten to derail your efforts discourage you. Focus on your progress and aim to protect the time and effort you have invested.

Control Cravings

Cravings are the extreme desire for a particular food. Expect to be visited by cravings and recognize that cravings are different from hunger. Hunger is the physical need to eat. Cravings are thought to be the result of complicated interactions of our senses, brain, and the gut-brain interactions.

You may want to eat but not really need to eat. Conversely, when you are hungry your body needs food but if you have lost your appetite (e.g. due to stress or fatigue) you may not want to eat. Ask yourself if you need to eat it because you are hungry or you want to eat it to make you feel good. If the answer is both, choose healthful food to satisfy your hunger.

You may discover that cravings will go away if you can ignore them, so actively employ strategies to put them off. For example, engage in physical activity, or occupy your mind with activities that are distracting, interesting and rewarding[265]. If you must satisfy cravings eat whole fruits or vegetables that fill you up and make it easier to ignore the cravings. It also helps not to have foods your crave within sight or readily available. Do keep fruits and vegetables within sight or readily available.

Fuhrman reports that a diet high in micronutrients appears to decrease food cravings and overeating behaviors[266]. Study participants who changed to a high nutrient density diet experience uncomfortable sensations of hunger less often than they experienced on their previous usual diet.

There is a lot to be said for variety. Studies have suggested that increasing the variety of healthful foods may help reduce food cravings in men but not women[267] and children experience stronger cravings than adults but they can also effectively regulate their cravings[268]. Consider the plight of rapacious birds:

"Many rapacious birds feed on one type of food and thus are wholly dependent on it, and they would go to the extremes of hunger before they would turn to another food source. Thus their habitat and distribution depends greatly on the prey available and their means of obtaining it."[269]

Don't waste your time and energy seeking foods you crave. Curb your rapacious appetite! Regardless of your age or sex, make variety an important element of your diet.

Studies show that you may reduce sugar cravings by including plant based fat and protein in your meals, eating cooked leafy greens, and getting eight hours sleep. Short sleep had been shown to reduce leptin and elevate ghrelin. Leptin is a hormone that suppresses appetite. Ghrelin is a stomach-derived hormone that stimulates appetite and its production increases with time since the last meal. Such differences in leptin and ghrelin are thought to increase appetite[270]. Also avoid getting too much protein in your diet, or at least more than you need. One complete protein source a day is enough.

Be prepared to address the issues posed by new comfort foods. Our brains are wired to repeat behaviors that feel good, so new eating habits can create new comfort foods too. For example, an aspiring vegetarian got in the habit of eating a huge dinner salad slowly while watching TV. After eating the salad over a period of 40-45 minutes, she craved steak, chicken, or fish, but decide instead on a small sandwich created with delicious plant-based chicken and cheese substitutes bundled in a whole grain wrap with salsa. Over time as she ate similar two course meals, the huge salad, which once represented over 90% of your caloric intake was reduced to 50% or less. And the increased intake was reflected in the weight she regained. Perhaps a wiser choice might have been to add to the huge salad, some pieces of salmon or strips of plant-based chicken substitutes, and include tomato chunks in the salad dressing, all the while maintaining the vegetables' 90% share of the total caloric intake.

Maintain an awareness of your caloric intake and limit your daily totals so that you don't exceed the calories needed to maintain your current weight. If you are gaining weight, you might be addicted to food.

Diet and Sleep Tradeoffs

Researchers have found that simple manipulation of food intake can significantly improve sleep. One study found a carbohydrate-based high-GI meal resulted in a significant shortening sleep onset[271]. Another study showed the consumption of a meal with a high-GI in the evening was associated with longer sleep duration[272]. And a third study found that a diet with a high-glycemic index is associated with good sleep quality[273]. However, although intakes of starchy foods like white rice with high GI contribute to good sleep, such diets are also reported to be associated with several health problems including obesity, diabetes mellitus, cardiovascular disease, and some cancers.

People with reflux symptoms and disorders (acid reflux, gastric reflux, indigestion, heartburn) should eat a light dinner and finish it at least 3 hours before going to bed. Late eating is a crucial risk factor for reflux. Salty foods, caffeinated beverages, and too much wine could contribute to poor sleep[274].

Standing the Pyramid on its Head

When asked to compare conventional processed food with vegan processed food, some writers used the expression "processed food is processed food," meaning they are equally to be avoided. Carefully reading and comparing labels show that is clearly not true. Processing per se is not harmful – compare freezing and frying food for example. Or butter and almond butter. Processed products with trans fat, added sugar, and sodium can be unhealthy. Healthful processed products do have a place on plant based food pyramids. They can be valuable resources during the transition period to help you avoid comfort foods and unhealthful processed meat and cheese. However, be mindful of the limits placed on processed foods by virtue of the space they occupy on your pyramid.

An alternative feasible strategy for the transition to a plant based diet is to build your meal from plant based processed food products with the same tastes and textures of familiar animal based foods that you are accustomed to eating. That approach turns the food pyramid upside down. And there are very few, if any, plant-based products that are indistinguishable from the poultry, beef, or fish products they were designed to imitate. While there are many commercial products to try, including a growing number of very good imitations, you can expect many disappointing experiences if you are seeking indistinguishable substitutes. Moreover, this strategy could lead to frustration, delay the transition, and might ultimately result in abandonment of the healthful diet. Additionally, excessive consumption of undesirable additives in the processed food would not be healthful.

It is probably more productive to accept the compromise of experiencing new tastes of healthful foods that are not expected to taste better than familiar food but are pleasing enough to grow to enjoy over time as your tastes change. In the event you find some plant-based processed products to be even more appealing than the familiar foods to which you were accustomed be sure to limit consumption to the allotment on your pyramid, or better yet, focus on the base and lower tiers, or try to transition to a totally whole foods, plant food based diet.

Cooking

Cooking doesn't just make foods taste better, it increases the energy available from foods. Don't be discouraged if you haven't yet learned to cook. According to a recent study even chimpanzees possess the suite of cognitive capacities required for cooking[275].

Lack of cooking knowledge, confidence, experience, and skills can limit at-home preparation of healthy meals. To learn to cook, begin by searching online, browsing recipe books and magazines at stores, or asking friends or relatives for palatable recipes with healthful ingredients.

Carefully read the recipes to be sure you understand them and have the means to follow them, even if you have to acquire some kitchen gadgets or substitute for some ingredients. Line up all of the ingredients to be sure that you know where they are when you need them and have sufficient quantities for the recipe. Don't be caught by surprise by the next instruction that calls for marinating the mixture overnight. Visualize how you are going to perform each step in the process, and think about any time constraints that might cause problems. For example, is it possible to clean and slice all of the mushrooms, peel and mince the garlic, and dice the onions in the eight minute window you have available before the next step in the recipe? Or will you have all of the necessary ingredients readily available to quickly blend them into a sauce that has to be removed from the burner within two minutes?

Cooking mistakes are common even among experts. Flavors or textures can be out of balance or unappealing. Recipes don't always call for the kinds or amounts of seasoning and ingredients you prefer; the preparation process can be faulty, the estimated cooking time might not be accurate, and results vary depending on the quality of your ingredients, your kitchen equipment, culinary experience and many other factors. To paraphrase Helen Keller:

Excellent cooking cannot be achieved without diligent trial and error. Nerve-wracking, humbling experience creates clear vision, inspires ambition, and leads to successful achievements.

Always approach a new recipe with the mindset of how to improve it. For instance, if the salad dressing recipe is too thick, double the volume of fluids or reduce or substitute for the solids. Build a notebook (online or hard copy) of recipes and work on improving them. Use your notebook to create your own cookbook whether you intend to publish it or not.

Substitution of ingredients in recipes, particularly those that require baking, is frowned upon because the results can be disastrous. However, that is a risk you might have to accept. If possible, try to find out if the substitution is likely to compromise the results.

Try not to cook things too long or too hot because those mistakes are irreversible and can be messy. Be especially careful not to over toast nuts and overcook vegetables. On the other hand, be aware that a hot pan is essential for sautéing and browning vegetables, and undercooked (or over kneaded) baked goods are not palatable. Allow sufficient time and the correct heat settings to caramelize vegetables. Be careful not to microwave what is not supposed to be microwaved, e.g. plastic containers that might contain BPA. Stir as long and often as the recipe suggests, and don't leave food unattended too long.

Overcrowd pots and frying pans can produce soggy products and vegetables will fail to caramelize. Choose fresh, high quality fruits and vegetables. Avoid the temptation of saving money on discounted food that is near its expiration date. Don't buy fish products that smell fishy or use refrigerated greens that have a foul odor. Carefully wash and dry salad greens; serving them on chilled plates will enhance their flavors. Do not wash lettuce until you are ready to use it, and store it just barely moist in the refrigerator at the correct humidity. Alternate between chopped and tossed salads to create more variety. Cook rice with plenty of water, like spaghetti, to avoid stickeyness. To avoid soggy pizza or flatbreads, use a pre-heated pan or pizza stone to bake a veggie pizza/flatbread that has been topped with previously sautéed vegetable toppings[276].

When the dish you prepare doesn't meet your expectations, try to determine what went wrong. If the errors might have been due to the recipe, use another recipe or modify the recipe to address the problems. Attempt to improve the recipes until you have achieved complete satisfaction. Then try to make it even better.

Your knowledge, confidence, and skills will grow with experience. Take advantage of opportunities to continue your education in various ways, e.g. train yourself to identify tastes and odors of spices and other ingredients and use that knowledge to modify your recipes. And experiment by tasting unfamiliar foods. Ask friends and relatives to critique the meals you prepare. Consider taking cooking classes, or give someone a gift of a hands-on cooking and dining class at a cooking school, instead of trying to find suitable food and entertainment at the buffet of a dinner theater.

Dessert

What about desserts? Try eating fruits for desserts. Among the sweetest are dates, figs, grapes, bananas, mangos, sweet cherries, apples, pineapples, and pears. But choose low-carbohydrate fruit and restrict the serving size (e.g. 15 grams of carbohydrates) if you are overweight or insulin resistant[277].

Is dark chocolate candy a healthy food? Studies claim that flavonoids — specifically catechin, epicatechin, and procyanidins – in cocoa can be healthy, but the high-calorie chocolate bars that contain sugar, milk, and other ingredients aren't necessarily good for you[278]. Limiting your dessert to very small servings of candy bars with very high cocoa content may not satisfy your appetite, but remember that your taste buds can be trained to enjoy foods with less-sweet flavor over time.

If you are overweight, try not to think about dessert.

Weight and Exercise

In Chapter Two we said it is important to monitor your weight during the period when you are changing your eating habits so that you can control your consumption of calories. And you can learn to control your weight by monitoring the pattern of weight changes and adjusting ("titrating") your eating, drinking, resting, and exercise routines. We suggested that monitoring daily weight changes might also help motivate you stay the course.

During the transition period, try to estimate the caloric values of your food choices and maintain an awareness of your daily caloric budget. Once you are habituated to a plant based diet you can expect to see little fluctuations in daily weight.

One theory about regaining lost weight is that people who decrease their caloric intake to lose weight experience a drop in their metabolic rate, making it increasingly difficult to lose weight. A lower metabolic rate may also make it easier to regain weight after a normal diet is resumed[279].

A 2003 report noted that studies of human subjects indicated a short-term elevation in resting metabolic rate in response to single exercise events. The elevation in resting metabolic rate appeared to have two phases, one lasting less than 2 hours and a smaller much more prolonged effect lasting up to 48 hours. And while many studies have shown that long-term training increases resting metabolic rate, many other studies failed to find such effects. Some of the studies concerning long-term effects of training were distorted by errors with the study designs. The long-term effects of training included increases in resting metabolic rate due to increases in lean muscle mass. Extreme interventions, however, may have induced reductions in resting metabolic rate, in spite of the increased lean tissue mass[280].

There's no easy way to lose weight. Dieting and exercise routines can be demotivating and there is a substantial risk of getting into a cycle of weight loss and weight regain, also known as yo-yoing. The same amount of caloric intake by groups of different people can result in different amounts and types of body fat in each group if, for example, one group is cycling their weights by dieting. You might not notice or mind losing muscle and gaining fat, but knowledge of the potentially dangerous and lasting effects may help keep you focused and maintain your resolve.

Yo-Yoing

Although there is still controversy whether weight cycling promotes body fat accumulation and obesity, many large-scale prospective studies have shown an association between weight fluctuations and cardiovascular morbidity and mortality. Higher prevalence of hypertension, accumulation of visceral fat, insulin resistance and dyslipidemia are more likely to occur in weight cyclers of normal body weight and may all contribute to cardiovascular risks. In addition, fluctuations of cardiovascular risk variables, such as blood pressure, heart rate, sympathetic activity, blood glucose and lipids, with probable repeated overshoots above normal values during periods of weight regain, put an additional stress on the cardiovascular system[281]. If you lose weight don't gain it back.

Exercise is effective for maintaining weight loss. Studies show that people who lose weight and keep it off over the long term get regular physical activity[282]. Running, cycling, swimming, using exercise equipment, and activities like hiking, dancing, and yard work can help you burn calories. Stay hydrated before, during, and after exercise. Drink water to stay hydrated and help reduce cravings. Avoid sweeteners and don't drink diet beverages. Add lemon or lime to your water or tea. Your appetite may increase after exercise. Eat mindfully, satisfy your appetite with nutrient dense whole foods instead of energy dense liquids.

Try to check your weight each morning. Cut back on your caloric intake for that day if you see a significant increase in weight or observe a slow steady climb to new morning weight highs.

Support

Many magazines, books, and blogs lead their readers to believe that the transition to a plant based diet is a cake walk. An uphill climb is a better metaphor. As we noted in the Preface the transition to a plant based diet will require great resolve and perseverance. Your journey will not be always smooth and uneventful but you need not row your boat alone. The people you work with, live with, and socialize with can have a huge impact on your diet style. They can offer encouragement and motivational support to keep moving forward and allow you to achieve a perspective on how well you are progressing.

If could also be very helpful if you recruit others to adopt a healthful eating lifestyle. You can share your experiences, suggest new ways of dealing with shared problems, and vent your stresses. You might even coach others and provide helpful hints based on your own experiences. A sense of community will enable all of you to give and receive support and help care for each other. Your companions cannot take your place at the helm but they can ensure that it is not a lonely journey.

Consider joining a food-coop. Co-ops are owned and governed by member-shoppers[283]. They can offer the benefits of organic, local produce. Some provide cooking classes, gardening lessons, monthly grocery baskets, and other community perks to their members.

Do not rely exclusively on others to provide motivation. Create your own feedback loop from your successful experiences including shopping, finding new restaurants, preparing delicious meals for yourself and others, and experiencing improvements in your health status (e.g. more stamina, less pain, no more headaches, etc.) that results from your transition to a plant based diet style.

If you have an entrepreneurial spirit, explore networking possibilities that might lead to business ventures that are associated with plant based products[284].

<u>Staying Informed</u>

At this point the reader should be able to address questions such as: Why all the confusion about milk, meat, fat, fish, etc. Why is it so difficult to get valid information? But you will have to remain vigilant. Continue to ask, "Who and what can I believe?"

Flip-flopping nutritional science announcements can also be demotivating, as well as annoying. Moreover, the burden of trying to determine whether nutritional science announcements are valid or important is likely to continue to test the patience of the public.

However, staying informed may help keep you motivated. Making the effort to determine the basis and validity of announcements might be helpful. For example, when nutrition authorities proclaimed that reducing saturated fat and trans fat in the diet was a better strategy than restricting foods that contain higher amounts of cholesterol, such as eggs, shrimp, and lobster, it was viewed by many as just another dietary flip-flop and tended to undermine their confidence in what is known about healthy eating. However, upon learning the basis for the new recommendations – namely, that cholesterol in food has little effect on the amount of cholesterol in the bloodstream, while saturated fat and trans fat in the diet damages blood vessels, which sets off the steady growth of plaque that can rupture and lead to heart attacks – it was easier for some people to regard the announcement as a sign of continuing progress and accept the recommendations[285].

For the foreseeable future there is not much anyone will do to change the confusing nature of nutritional science pronouncement. But don't get discouraged, there are a number of incisive questions to ask about the claims and announcements to help you determine their credibility and how important the results are for you personally.

The Harvard School of Public Health published five quick tips for putting health news in context:

1. *Is the story simply reporting the results of a single study?* – the results of single studies are rarely sufficient to warrant changing people's behaviors.
2. *How large is the study?* – the results of large studies are often more reliable.
3. *Was the study done in animals or humans?* – additional studies must almost always be performed with human subjects. [note that humans are animals too]
4. *Did the study look at real disease endpoints, like heart disease or osteoporosis?* – disease endpoints might not occur for decades, and results based only on markers for the diseases may turn out not be valid.
5. *How was diet assessed?* – good studies will furnish evidence that the methods were valid[286].

There are many other appropriate, incisive questions that can be asked, but the answers will frequently not be readily available. So as is often the case in life, people have to make decisions with whatever information is available. Some other questions to ask include:

Did you learn of the findings from the publication of the original source? – if it was from an article in a newspaper, magazine, website, or a broadcast on radio or TV, you should examine the original source before acting on the results[287].

How current is the information? – outdated information can be misleading or dangerous especially if the information has been superseded or discredited.

Who funded the study? – a study about diet supplements funded by the manufacturer of diet supplements should be viewed with the same skepticism as their advertisements; a study funded by a government agency with stakeholders who influence their policies may have even less credence; government funding is subject to politics and policy reviews that can be subtle but heavy handed; university studies funded by an organizations with vested interests in the outcomes are also suspect; organizational conflicts of interest are widespread but often not evident.

Do the authors or the editors, or publishers have conflicting interests? – studies have found correlations with results benefiting sponsors, poor study design, withholding negative data from publication, and other problems[288]; to deal with Investigators' outside financial interests and promote transparency, some universities require disclosure of related financial interests in publications and presentations. Some journals also require such disclosures.

What are the credentials of the authors? – Thomas Edison and Michael Faraday did not have formal educations. Reliable and useful information is often reported in articles written by people who don't list impressive credentials. But the information that you rely on should be described correctly and referenced so that it can be validated. It is very important to check all dietary health information you see published by an individual's of unknown credentials. Some articles contain good information but also contain myths or rumors. And the statements of the authors frequently do not correctly describe what is being attributed to the referenced sources.

What do others say about the announcement? – search for reports by two or more independent experts concerning the study. Look for research or papers that cite the announcement and be aware of the credentials, affiliations, and conflicts of interest of those citing the announcement. Citation databases exist that are supposed to make it possible to search cited references; that is, they search for references that are listed in the bibliographies of research publications. Users can follow a particular cited reference, or cited author, forward in time to find other articles that have also cited that author or work.

What types of research methods were used and what are their limitations? – are the findings based on laboratory animal studies or people? – were the people in the study of a similar age, sex, education level, income group, and ethnic background as you? – was the results from a randomized controlled clinical trial or an observational study? – was the research performed at one institution or by a coordinated effort involving studies at several institutions? – were the results merely statistically significant or significant enough to actually be important?[289]

Are the reported results consistent with previous studies? – if the results are very different from previous published studies they must be independently validated by other researchers. Significantly different results need to be repeated elsewhere several times before they might be considered truly valid.

Have any potential interactions with other substances, side effects, and unintended consequences been investigated? – new supplements or proposed dietary changes might create or worsen an existing health problem. Ask yourself what are the consequences of acting on the information; if there are potential health risks seek advice from a physician you can trust.

Did the author clearly communicate the findings of the research? – the study should state concisely what can be concluded and its implications as in the following example:

"The evidence to date suggests that dietary calcium does not increase CVD risk and may even reduce risk. However, the majority of data regarding the relationship between calcium intake and CVD risk has been extrapolated from observational studies. Results are inherently limited because of design flaws, including the possible presence of confounding factors, recall bias, inability to accurately determine causality, and researcher bias in outcome assessment. Results from the few RCTs are mixed regarding CVD risk in those using supplemental calcium with or without vitamin D, although the majority of studies found no increased risk. This question still remains to be more definitively answered by large-scale, randomized trials designed specifically with CVD as the primary end point. Available evidence suggests that if there is a risk, it is more likely to be attributed to calcium supplementation alone. Larger and longer RCTs are needed to confirm this association, although these trials may be economically challenging to conduct. The utility of calcium supplementation is still being debated, yet evidence suggests that it is reasonable to

encourage adequate dietary calcium intake, especially for postmenopausal women who are at greatest risk for osteoporotic fracture."[290]

Interestingly, a recent systematic review and meta-analysis to determine whether increasing calcium intake from dietary sources affects bone mineral density (BMD) and whether the effects are similar to those of calcium supplements concluded increasing calcium intake from dietary sources increases BMD by a similar amount to increases in BMD from calcium supplements. However, *"the small effects on BMD are unlikely to translate into clinically meaningful reductions in fractures. Therefore, for most individuals concerned about their bone density, increasing calcium intake is unlikely to be beneficial."*[291]

Finally, even if you are satisfied with the answers to those questions, you need to be aware of your own biases especially when reading articles that say things that you agree with but might also contain biased statements that are not valid.

A large and growing number of people use the Internet for information and advice on dietary and nutritional information. We believe that the number has surpassed the number who use print and broadcast media as their major sources of nutrition information. While statistics are lacking for North America, an Australian study found that the use of the Internet as a main source of nutrition information grew rapidly since 2004, with one-third of Western Australian adults reported using the Internet for that purpose in 2012[292].

With the growing popularity of the Internet, it has become easier and faster to access nutrition and health information. However, you should be aware that all information placed on the internet is unregulated. Hence, the Internet also allows rapid and widespread distribution of false and misleading nutrition and health information.

All of the aforementioned questions and considerations concerning the credibility and importance of claims and announcements apply to Internet sources and there are several additional suggestions that may prove to be helpful as well:

Many online resources are useful, but others may present information that is inaccurate or misleading, so it's important to find sources you can trust and to know how to evaluate their content.
Look for an *"About Us"* page. Check to see who runs the site: Is it a branch of the government, a university, a health organization, a hospital or a business? Can you trust them? Does the site have an editorial board? Is the information reviewed before it is posted? Look for the names and credentials of the individuals who reviewed a Web page in an Acknowledgments section near the end of the page.

You want current, unbiased information based on <u>research</u>. When was the information posted or reviewed? Is it up-to-date? Where did the information come from? Is it based on scientific research? If the person or organization in charge of the site didn't create the material, the original source should be clearly identified.

What is the purpose of the site? Is it selling something? Who pays for the Web site? Do the claims seem too good to be true?[293]

You can sometimes find accurate health information quickly and easily starting with one of these organized collections of up-to-date resources:

>MedlinePlus, sponsored by the National Library of Medicine, which is part of the National Institutes of Health (NIH) (use this link: https://www.nlm.nih.gov/medlineplus/)
>PubMed® to search MEDLINE® for citations to professional medical literature.
>NLM PubMed Health for clinical effectiveness research information.
>PubMed Central® (PMC) to search a free archive of biomedical and life sciences journal literature at the NLM.

For guidance on how to evaluate the information that you find see:

>MedlinePlus Evaluating Internet Health Information, National Library of Medicine
>Evaluating Online Sources of Health Information, NIH National Cancer Institute
>How to Evaluate Health Information on the Internet, NIH Office of Dietary Supplements
>A User's Guide to Finding and Evaluating Health Information on the Web, Medical Library Association

(Or use the link found at endnote number 294 in the References[294])

In closing we caution the reader to be mindful of the widespread under appreciation among scientists and policymakers regarding the limitations of observational data for establishing cause-effect relations between dietary exposures and health outcomes[295]. It is important to remain aware that conclusions based on observational research should be regarded with caution. Observational studies cannot prove that an association reflects cause and effect. We leave you with this poem which has served to help many researchers who were intrigued by observations to avoid the pitfalls of misinterpretation. It is John Godfrey Saxe's (1816-1887) version of the famous Indian legend:

>It was six men of Indostan
>To learning much inclined,
>Who went to see the Elephant
>(Though all of them were blind),
>That each by observation
>Might satisfy his mind.
>
>The First approach'd the Elephant,
>And happening to fall
>Against his broad and sturdy side,
>At once began to bawl:
>"God bless me! but the Elephant
>Is very like a wall!"

The Second, feeling of the tusk,
Cried, -"Ho! what have we here
So very round and smooth and sharp?
To me 'tis mighty clear
This wonder of an Elephant
Is very like a spear!"

The Third approached the animal,
And happening to take
The squirming trunk within his hands,
Thus boldly up and spake:
"I see," quoth he, "the Elephant
Is very like a snake!"

The Fourth reached out his eager hand,
And felt about the knee.
"What most this wondrous beast is like
Is mighty plain," quoth he,
"'Tis clear enough the Elephant
Is very like a tree!"

The Fifth, who chanced to touch the ear,
Said: "E'en the blindest man
Can tell what this resembles most;
Deny the fact who can,
This marvel of an Elephant
Is very like a fan!"

The Sixth no sooner had begun
About the beast to grope,
Then, seizing on the swinging tail
That fell within his scope,
"I see," quoth he, "the Elephant
Is very like a rope!"

And so these men of Indostan
Disputed loud and long,
Each in his own opinion
Exceeding stiff and strong,
Though each was partly in the right,
And all were in the wrong!

Please explore the references in Chapter Ten and good luck with your delicious, healthful journey.

Chapter Ten: Satisfying Your Appetite for Knowledge

Every day, everywhere there are things being said and written about food. The sheer mass of information that has been created is beyond compilation. The daily additions (e.g. with new menus, new products, new articles, new restaurants, etc.) are creating a massive jumble of facts, judgments, opinions, fiction, lies, etc. There doesn't seem to be any single credible source untainted by self-interest, politics, corruption, ignorance, etc. It is "every man for himself."

It is feasible for a layperson to become knowledgeable about major food and health issues but to actually be well-informed on a scientific issue, you have to read an enormous body of peer-reviewed literature.

This final chapter lists references to articles on a variety of topics that are discussed in the book. URLs are provided to allow access to articles published on the Internet. With a few exceptions, they are available online at no cost.

Preface

http://time.com/3929990/americans-overweight-obese/
Dawn Jackson Blatner, The Flexitarian Diet: The Mostly Vegetarian Way to Lose Weight, Be Healthier, Prevent Disease, and Add Years to Your Life, McGraw-Hill, 2008.
http://www.webmd.com/diet/a-z/flexitarian_diet?page=2
http://www.ijhssnet.com/journals/Vol_1_No_12_September_2011/12.pdf
http://consumewithcare.org/the-rise-of-the-flexitarian/
Fuhrman, Joel, The End of Dieting: How to live for life, New York, NY: HarperOne, 2014.
  http://www.ncbi.nlm.nih.gov/pmc/articles/PMC3342754/

Chapter One

Carpenter, Kenneth J. 2003, "A Short History of Nutritional Science: Part 1 (1785–1885)," Journal of Nutrition 133: 638-645. http://jn.nutrition.org/content/133/3/638.full.pdf
Carpenter, Kenneth J. 2003, "A Short History of Nutritional Science: Part 2 (1885–1912)," Journal of Nutrition 133: 975-984. http://jn.nutrition.org/content/133/4/975.full.pdf
Carpenter, Kenneth J. 2003, "A Short History of Nutritional Science: Part 3 (1912–1944)," Journal of Nutrition 133: 3023-3032. http://jn.nutrition.org/content/133/10/3023.full.pdf
Carpenter, Kenneth J. 2003, "A Short History of Nutritional Science: Part 4 (1945–1985)," Journal of Nutrition 133: 3331-3342. http://jn.nutrition.org/content/133/11/3331.full.pdf
http://www.pnas.org/content/111/16/5773.full
http://www.sciencedaily.com/releases/2008/12/081202133513.htm
https://hbr.org/2014/03/when-research-should-come-with-a-warning-label/
http://www.uniteforsight.org/global-health-university/nutrition-study
http://people.vetmed.wsu.edu/jmgay/courses/GlossClinStudy.htm
http://www.pccrp.org/docs/pccrp%20section%20i.pdf
http://www.acog.org/Resources-And-Publications/Department-Publications/Reading-the-Medical-Literature

http://wayback.archive.org/web/20060219042545/http://www.economics.soton.ac.uk/staff/aldrich/spurious.pdf
Aldrich, John, "Correlations Genuine and Spurious in Pearson and Yule," Statistical Science 10 (4): 364–376.
http://www.ncbi.nlm.nih.gov/pubmed/8261254
Fleiss J,L, "The statistical basis of meta-analysis," Statistical Methods in Medical Research, 1993; 2(2):121-45.
https://academics.utep.edu/portals/321/faculty%20pages/cohn/how%20meta-analysis%20increases%20statistical%20power.pdf
Cohn, Lawrence D, and Betsy J. Becker, "How Meta-Analysis Increases Statistical Power," Psychological Methods, 2003, Vol. 8, No. 3, 243–253.
https://www.nia.nih.gov/health/publication/understanding-risk
http://oregonstate.edu/ua/ncs/archives/2013/dec/review-most-clinical-studies-vitamins-flawed-poor-methodology
http://www.realclearscience.com/blog/2013/10/40-years-of-government-nutrition-data-may-be-flawed.html
http://news.sciencemag.org/health/2014/03/scientists-fix-errors-controversial-paper-about-saturated-fats
http://www.eurekalert.org/pub_releases/2013-10/uosc-4yo100913.php
http://www.eufic.org/article/en/expid/understaninhttp://tierneylab.blogs.nytimes.com/2007/11/01/is-nutrition-science-not-really-science/?_r=0g-scientific-studies/
http://www.geneticliteracyproject.org/2014/07/15/study-claiming-organic-food-more-nutritious-deeply-flawed-say-independent-scientists/
http://ajcn.nutrition.org/content/90/6/1700.full
http://www.ncbi.nlm.nih.gov/pubmed/20184991
http://jacknorrisrd.com/nutrition-research-what-you-should-know/
http://www.veganhealth.org/articles/dxrates
http://scholarlykitchen.sspnet.org/2012/07/18/a-proposed-list-60-things-journal-publishers-do/
http://www.nytimes.com/2014/02/09/opinion/sunday/why-nutrition-is-so-confusing.html?_r=0http://www.foodandnutritionresearch.net/index.php/fnr/article/viewFile/1765/1672
http://www.npr.org/sections/health-shots/2015/06/09/413140503/costs-of-slipshod-research-methods-may-be-in-the-billions

Chapter Two

http://arbl.cvmbs.colostate.edu/hbooks/pathphys/endocrine/basics/chem.html
https://www.boundless.com/biology/textbooks/boundless-biology-textbook/the-endocrine-system-37/types-of-hormones-210/lipid-derived-amino-acid-derived-and-peptide-hormones-793-12028/
http://www.nature.com/nutd/journal/v2/n1/full/nutd201121a.html
http://neuroscience.mssm.edu/nestler/brainRewardpathways.html
https://www.jstage.jst.go.jp/article/endocrj/57/5/57_K10E-077/_pdf
http://www.iffgd.org/site/gi-disorders/digestive-system
http://www.precisionnutrition.com/all-about-appetite-1
http://www.psyking.net/id36.htm
http://themedicalbiochemistrypage.org/gut-brain.php
http://bk.psu.edu/clt/bisc4/ipweb/misc/assignmentfiles/digestive/Control.pdf
http://www.ncbi.nlm.nih.gov/books/NBK279994/

https://www.boundless.com/physiology/textbooks/boundless-anatomy-and-physiology-textbook/the-digestive-system-23/chemical-digestion-224/chemical-digestion-of-carbohydrates-proteins-lipids-and-nucleic-acids-1104-1171/
http://www.innerbody.com/image/digeov.html
http://www.nhlbi.nih.gov/files/docs/guidelines/ob_gdlns.pdf
http://www.wholefoodsmarket.com/healthy-eating/andi-guide
http://blog.lifeextension.com/2011/11/most-nutrient-dense-foods.html
http://ajcn.nutrition.org/content/95/4/989.full
http://www.ncbi.nlm.nih.gov/pmc/articles/PMC2897177/
http://www.mayoclinic.org/healthy-lifestyle/weight-loss/in-depth/metabolism/art-20046508?pg=2
http://www.precisionnutrition.com/all-about-energy-balance
http://www.bodyrecomposition.com/fat-loss/the-energy-balance-equation.html/
http://www.nature.com/ijo/journal/v35/n2s/pdf/ijo201169a.pdf?origin=publication_detail
http://circ.ahajournals.org/content/126/1/126.full
http://www.ncbi.nlm.nih.gov/pubmed/7315785
http://www.ncbi.nlm.nih.gov/pubmed/10435656
http://depts.washington.edu/uwcphn/news/presentations/NRF_041609.pdf
http://ajcn.nutrition.org/content/99/5/1223S.long
http://www.4er.org/CourseNotes/Book%20A/A-I.pdf
http://ajcn.nutrition.org/content/82/4/721.long
http://www.openhealthnews.com/blogs/groenpj/2011-10-05/nutrition-diet-free-open-source-andor-low-cost-solutions
http://www.uml.edu/campusrecreation/staff/EP%20II%20Materials/BC%20Lab.pdf
http://www.ncbi.nlm.nih.gov/pubmed/21085903
http://www.ncbi.nlm.nih.gov/pubmed/18517106
http://www.nap.edu/catalog.php?record_id=21654
http://themedicalbiochemistrypage.org/gut-brain.php
http://www.ncbi.nlm.nih.gov/pmc/articles/PMC1986582/
http://www.ncbi.nlm.nih.gov/pmc/articles/PMC2710609/
http://www.ncbi.nlm.nih.gov/pubmed/25534419
http://nrc.ajums.ac.ir/_nrc/documents/Molecular%20Basis%20of%20Human%20Nutrition.pdf
http://www.health.harvard.edu/blog/why-eating-slowly-may-help-you-feel-full-faster-20101019605
https://www.drfuhrman.com/library/andi-food-scores.aspx
http://ajcn.nutrition.org/content/82/4/721.full

Chapter Three

http://www.superfoodsrx.com/healthyliving/low-fat-foods-dont-be-fooled-by-fat-labels/
http://www.fda.gov/Food/IngredientsPackagingLabeling/LabelingNutrition/ucm20026097.htm
http://www.fda.gov/ForConsumers/ConsumerUpdates/ucm094536.htm
http://www.fda.gov/Food/GuidanceRegulation/GuidanceDocumentsRegulatoryInformation/LabelingNutrition/ucm064928.htm
http://www.fda.gov/Food/IngredientsPackagingLabeling/LabelingNutrition/ucm274593.htm
http://www.heart.org/HEARTORG/GettingHealthy/NutritionCenter/HealthyEating/Understanding-Food-Nutrition-Labels_UCM_300132_Article.jsp#.VibzrH6rTDc
http://www.health.com/health/gallery/0,,20708150,00.html
http://www.diabetes.org/food-and-fitness/food/what-can-i-eat/food-tips/taking-a-closer-look-at-labels.html?referrer=https://www.google.com/

http://www.mayoclinic.org/healthy-lifestyle/nutrition-and-healthy-eating/multimedia/reading-food-labels/flh-20078339
http://www.naturalnews.com/021929_groceries_food_products.html#ixzz3o0LDBcM6
http://www.huffingtonpost.com/2013/06/22/how-read-food-label_n_3472529.html
http://www.scp-knowledge.eu/sites/default/files/knowledge/attachments/Hieke_Taylor_2012_Review%20Nutritional%20Labeling.pdf
http://www.cnn.com/2015/01/14/health/feat-natural-flavors-explained/
http://www.today.com/food/food-q-just-what-natural-flavoring-2D80554450

Chapter Four

http://www.huffingtonpost.com/2014/01/31/best-comfort-food_n_4698104.html
http://www.foodnetwork.com/recipes/photos/americas-best-top-10-comfort-foods.html
http://www.southernliving.com/food/classic-comfort-food-recipes
http://www.buzzfeed.com/emofly/best-comfort-foods-ever#.wrj96oVwa
http://www.ncbi.nlm.nih.gov/pubmed/24105325
http://www.ncbi.nlm.nih.gov/pmc/articles/PMC4311273/
http://ajcn.nutrition.org/content/86/4/895.full#fn-1
https://nccih.nih.gov/health/herbsataglance.htm
https://ods.od.nih.gov/HealthInformation/DS_WhatYouNeedToKnow.aspx
http://www.examiner.com/article/is-the-cinnamon-your-cupboard-an-imposter
https://cinnamonvogue.com/DOWNLOADS/Cinnamon_and_coumarin.pdf
http://thirtyseven.scientopia.org/tag/fda/
http://www.drugs.com/npp/cinnamon.html
http://www.care2.com/causes/theres-more-in-a-dash-of-cinnamon-than-you-might-care-to-know.html
http://www.wsj.com/articles/SB10001424052702303376904579135502891970942
http://thirtyseven.scientopia.org/2012/12/18/tis-the-season-for-cinnamon-or-is-it-cassia/
http://www.ncbi.nlm.nih.gov/pubmed/23627682
http://www.sciencedaily.com/releases/2010/11/101103135352.htm
http://www.theprairiehomestead.com/2013/11/will-the-real-cinnamon-please-stand-up.html
http://www.bfr.bund.de/en/faq_on_coumarin_in_cinnamon_and_other_foods-8487.html
https://hfnet.nih.go.jp/usr/soza1/BfR_061013_English.pdf
http://cinnamonvogue.com/DOWNLOADS/Cinnamon%20Side%20Effects.pdf
http://www.peoplespharmacy.com/2013/12/30/cinnamon-offers-health-benefits-but-also-carries-serious-risks/
http://healthyeating.sfgate.com/dangers-coumarin-cassia-cinnamon-11595.html
https://www.drfuhrman.com/library/choosing_the_right_cinnamon.aspx
http://www.ewg.org/research/how-much-is-too-much/harmful-effects-excess-vitamins-and-minerals
http://www.cmaj.ca/content/169/1/47.full
http://www.ncbi.nlm.nih.gov/pmc/articles/PMC164945/
http://www.mayoclinic.org/documents/mc5129-0709-sp-rpt-pdf/doc-20079085
http://www.hsph.harvard.edu/nutritionsource/salt-and-sodium/
http://archinte.jamanetwork.com/article.aspx?articleid=617252
http://pennstatehershey.adam.com/content.aspx?productId=117&pid=1&gid=000332
http://lpi.oregonstate.edu/mic/minerals/calcium#safety
http://health.clevelandclinic.org/2014/05/supplements-taking-many-can-hurt/
https://ods.od.nih.gov/factsheets/Iron-HealthProfessional/

http://lpi.oregonstate.edu/mic/minerals/magnesium
https://ods.od.nih.gov/factsheets/Magnesium-HealthProfessional/
https://umm.edu/health/medical/altmed/supplement/phosphorus
https://ods.od.nih.gov/factsheets/Selenium-HealthProfessional/
http://www.ncbi.nlm.nih.gov/pubmed/11967714
http://www.ncbi.nlm.nih.gov/pubmed/357085
http://lpi.oregonstate.edu/mic/minerals/sodium
https://www.heart.org/idc/groups/heart-public/@wcm/@hcm/documents/downloadable/ucm_300625.pdf
http://www.nhs.uk/Livewell/Goodfood/Pages/salt.aspx
http://www.fda.gov/ForConsumers/ConsumerUpdates/ucm181577.htm
http://www.washingtonpost.com/news/wonkblog/wp/2015/04/06/more-scientists-doubt-salt-is-as-bad-for-you-as-the-government-says/
http://lpi.oregonstate.edu/mic/minerals/sodium
https://ods.od.nih.gov/factsheets/Zinc-HealthProfessional/
http://lpi.oregonstate.edu/mic/minerals/zinc
http://www.nutri-facts.org/eng/trace-elements/zinc/safety/
http://www.arthritis.org/living-with-arthritis/treatments/natural/vitamins-minerals/too-many-vitamins-minerals.php
http://www.ift.org/~/media/Food%20Technology/pdf/2009/04/0409feat_NewColor.pdf
http://www.fda.gov/ForConsumers/ConsumerUpdates/ucm048951.htm
http://www.fda.gov/ForIndustry/ColorAdditives/RegulatoryProcessHistoricalPerspectives/
http://www.mayoclinic.org/diseases-conditions/adhd/expert-answers/adhd/faq-20058203
http://healthyeating.sfgate.com/sodium-nitrate-vs-sodium-nitrite-9064.html
http://www.accessdata.fda.gov/scripts/cdrh/cfdocs/cfCFR/CFRSearch.cfm?fr=172.175
http://www.fda.gov/ucm/groups/fdagov-public/@fdagov-foods-gen/documents/document/ucm269122.pdf
http://www.mayoclinic.org/healthy-lifestyle/nutrition-and-healthy-eating/expert-answers/sodium-nitrate/faq-20057848
http://www.foodproductdesign.com/topics/nitrates-nitrites.aspx
http://www.atsdr.cdc.gov/csem/csem.asp?csem=28&po=8
http://www.atsdr.cdc.gov/csem/nitrate_2013/docs/nitrite.pdf
http://fyi.uwex.edu/meats/files/2012/02/Nitrate-and-nitrite-in-cured-meat_10-18-2012.pdf
http://ajcn.nutrition.org/content/90/1/1.full
http://www.scribd.com/doc/262143221/Nitrates-Summary#scribd
http://www.hsph.harvard.edu/news/press-releases/processed-meats-unprocessed-heart-disease-diabetes/
http://ajpregu.physiology.org/content/early/2015/06/15/ajpregu.00099.2015
http://www.ncbi.nlm.nih.gov/pmc/articles/PMC3680013/
http://www.healthline.com/health/food-nutrition/is-sodium-nitrate-bad-for-you#3
http://pediatrics.aappublications.org/content/116/3/784.full.pdf
http://www.fsis.usda.gov/shared/PDF/Labeling_Requirements_Guide.pdf
http://www.medicaldaily.com/what-your-food-labeling-really-means-242823
http://www.accessdata.fda.gov/scripts/fcn/fcnNavigation.cfm?rpt=eafusListing&displayAll=true
http://www.fda.gov/Food/IngredientsPackagingLabeling/FoodAdditivesIngredients/ucm091048.htm
http://www.fda.gov/Food/IngredientsPackagingLabeling/ucm112642.htm
http://www.berkeleywellness.com/healthy-eating/food-safety/article/two-preservatives-avoid
http://www.efsa.europa.eu/en/efsajournal/pub/2588.htm
http://ntp.niehs.nih.gov/ntp/roc/content/profiles/butylatedhydroxyanisole.pdf

http://articles.chicagotribune.com/2013-01-21/news/ct-met-banned-food-additives-sidebar-20130121_1_potassium-bromate-flour-probable-carcinogen
http://articles.chicagotribune.com/2013-01-21/news/ct-met-banned-food-additives-sidebar-20130121_1_potassium-bromate-flour-probable-carcinogen

Chapter Five

http://www.med.upenn.edu/biocbiop/faculty/vanderkooi/chap7-9.pdf
http://www.getvegucated.com/latests-challenges/mimicking-meat-tofu-tempeh-seitan/
https://my.clevelandclinic.org/health/diseases_conditions/hic_Diabetes_Basics/hic_Diet_and_Diabetes/hic_Flavoring_Foods_Without_Salt
http://www.wholefoodsmarket.com/healthy-eating/add-flavor-naturally
http://umm.edu/health/medical/altmed/supplement/omega6-fatty-acids
http://www.mayoclinic.org/diseases-conditions/heart-disease/expert-answers/omega-6/faq-20058172

Chapter Six

http://thesweethome.com/reviews/best-kitchen-scale/
http://food-scales-review.toptenreviews.com/
http://www.goodhousekeeping.com/appliances/food-processor-reviews/
http://www.consumerreports.org/cro/food-processors-choppers.htm
http://www.consumersearch.com/food-processors
http://www.goodhousekeeping.com/cooking-tools/best-kitchen-knives/g646/best-kitchen-cutlery/
http://www.goodhousekeeping.com/health-products/bathroom-scale-reviews/a16776/bathroom-scales-tested/
http://www.myweighin.net/
http://blog.withings.com/2012/10/23/position-control-for-the-most-accurate-weigh-ins/

Chapter Seven

http://www.rd.com/health/wellness/rethink-what-you-drink/5/#ixzz3k4OzCx00
http://www.cal-water.com/pdf/On-Water.pdf
http://www.splendidtable.org/story/how-make-homemade-tofu
http://www.huffingtonpost.com/2014/10/28/homemade-tofu_n_6058254.html
http://www.vrg.org/recipes/vjseitan.htm

Chapter Eight

http://www.peta.org/blog/top-eight-vegetarian-restaurants-america/
http://www.cnn.com/2014/06/06/travel/vegetarian-destinations/
http://www.thrillist.com/eat/nation/21-best-vegetarian-and-vegan-restaurants-in-america
http://www.thedailymeal.com/travel/top-25-vegetarian-restaurants-world

Chapter Nine

http://www.wikihow.com/Saut%C3%A9
http://www.cooksmarts.com/cs-blog/2014/10/add-flavor-aromatics/
http://chinesefood.about.com/library/blstirfrytips.htm

http://www.sparkpeople.com/resource/nutrition_articles.asp?id=297&page=2
http://www.vegetariantimes.com/article/ingredient-substitution-guide/
http://dish.allrecipes.com/common-ingredient-substitutions/
http://www.joyofbaking.com/IngredientSubstitution.html
http://www.hsph.harvard.edu/nutritionsource/muffin-makeover/
http://www.theguardian.com/lifeandstyle/wordofmouth/2013/feb/26/healthy-food-train-yourself-like-it

Appendix

PHYTOCHEMICALS INCLUDED IN ANDI SCORING

Phytosterols, plant-derived sterols similar in structure and function to cholesterol.

Glucosinolates, a large group of sulfur-containing compounds found in cruciferous vegetables. Food processing, chopping or chewing results in the release of the enzyme myrosinase. Myrosinase hydrolyzes glucosinolates to form isothiocyanates – isothiocyanates have been shown to inhibit human tumors cells. But *"much remains to be learned regarding cruciferous vegetable consumption and cancer prevention."*[296]

Angiogenesis inhibitors interfere with blood vessel formation. Angiogenesis, the process of the formation of new blood vessels from preexisting capillaries is a feature of numerous pathological conditions including: the growth of capillaries into the tumors leads to their enlargement and helps the tumor cells to metastasize; the formation of new blood vessels in the enlarging atherosclerotic plaque; the inflammatory synovium of the rheumatoid arthritic joints; some incurable skin diseases, particularly psoriasis.

Organosulfides found mostly in cruciferous vegetables, as well as garlic. Allium, sulforaphane, glutathione and isothiocyanates are organosulfides that are generally considered as beneficial for health because of their anti-carcinogenic, anti-thrombotic, anti-atherosclerotic, anti-inflammatory, anti-microbial and anti-oxidative effects.

Aromatase inhibitors (AIs) have been utilized as either anticancer agents or for cancer chemoprevention. Aromatase is an enzyme responsible for catalyzing the biosynthesis of estrogens (estrone and estradiol) from androgens (androstenedione and testosterone). Aromatase has been found in numerous tissues throughout the body including breast, skin, brain, adipose, muscle, and bone. The concentration of estrogens has been shown to be as much as twenty-fold higher in breast cancer tissues than in the circulating plasma, suggesting locally increased aromatase expression for estrogen biosynthesis near or within the cancerous tissues. Inhibition of the aromatase enzyme has been shown to reduce estrogen production throughout the body to nearly undetectable levels and is proving to have significant affect on the development and progression of hormone-responsive breast cancers. However, the use of AIs for cancer chemotherapy or chemoprevention is limited to postmenopausal women or premenopausal women who have undergone ovarian ablation[297].

Resistant starch is a term applied to the starch and starch degradation products that escape from digestion in the small intestine of healthy individuals. Resistant starch is considered a type of dietary fiber, because it can deliver some of the benefits of insoluble fiber and some of the benefits of soluble fiber.

Resveratrol is a polyphenolic compound naturally found in peanuts, grapes, red wine, and some berries. The bioavailability of resveratrol is relatively low because it is rapidly metabolized and eliminated. In preclinical studies, resveratrol has been shown to possess numerous biological functions, which could possibly be applied to the prevention and/or treatment of cancer, cardiovascular disease, and neurodegenerative diseases. Although resveratrol can inhibit the growth of cancer cells in culture and in some animal models, it is not known whether resveratrol can prevent and/or help treat cancer in humans[298].

ORAC stands for oxygen radical absorbance capacity. It is a laboratory test that attempts to quantify the total antioxidant capacity of food by measuring the ability of a food to quench oxygen free radicals in a test tube. ORAC is a somewhat controversial topic. The USCA has removed the ORAC Database from their website *"due to mounting evidence that the values indicating antioxidant capacity have no relevance to the effects of specific bioactive compounds, including polyphenols on human health."*[299]

ETHYLENE PRODUCTION AND SENSITIVITY OF PERISHABLE FRUITS & VEGETABLES

Perishable Fruits & Vegetables	Ethylene Production	Ethylene Sensitivity
Apple	Very High	High (Scald or Lose Crunch, Accelerate Senescence)
Apricot	High	High (Hastens Ripening, Decay)
Artichoke	Very Low	Low
Asian Pear	High	High (Accelerate Loss of Green Color, Increase Softening, Decay)
Asparagus	Very Low	Medium (Toughness)
Avocado (California)	High	High (Hastens Ripening)
Avocado (Tropical)	High	High (Hastens Ripening, Decay)
Banana	Medium	High (Hastens Ripening, Decay)
Beans (Lima)	Low	Medium (Loss of Green Pigment, Browning)
Beans (Snap/Green)	Low	Medium (Loss of Green Pigment, Browning)
Belgian Endive	Very Low	Medium
Berries	Low	Low (Mold)
Berries (Cranberry)	Low	Low (Mold)
Berries (Strawberry)	Low	Low (Mold)
Breadfruit	Medium	Medium
Broccoli	Very Low	High (Floret Yellowing)
Brussel Sprouts	Very Low	High (Yellowing)
Cabbage	Very Low	High (Leaf Abscission, Leaf Yellowing)
Cantalope	High	Medium (Over-Ripening, Decay)
Cape Gooseberry	Low	Low
Carrots (Topped)	Very Low	Low (Bitterness)
Casaba Melon	Low	Low
Cauliflower	Very Low	High (Discoloration of Curd, Accelerated Yellowing, Detachment of Wrapper Leaf Stalks)
Celery	Very Low	Medium (Loss of Green Color)
Chard	Very Low	High
Cherimoya	Very High	High (Accelerates Ripening, Decay)
Cherry (Sour)	Very Low	Low (Softening)
Cherry (Sweet)	Very Low	Low (Softening)
Chicory	Very Low	High
Chinese Gooseberry	Low	High
Collards	Very Low	Medium
Crenshaw Melon	Medium	High (Accelerates Ripening, Decay)
Cucumbers	Low	High (Yellowing)
Eggplant	Low	High (Calyx Abscission, Brown Spots, Increased Deterioration)
Endive (Escarole)	Very Low	Medium
Feijoa	Medium	Low
Figs	Medium	Low
Garlic	Very Low	Low (Odor)
Ginger	Very Low	Low
Grapefruit (AZ,CA,FL,TX)	Very Low	Medium (Mold)
Grapes	Very Low	Low (Mold)
Greens (Leafy)	Very Low	High (Russet Spotting)
Guava	Low	Medium
Honeydew	Medium	High (Accelerates Ripening, Decay)
Jack Fruit	Medium	Medium (Accelerates Ripening, Decay)
Kale	Very Low	Medium
Kiwi Fruit	Low	High (Induces Softening, Decay)
Leeks	Very Low	Medium
Lemons	Very Low	High (Mold)

Lettuce (Butterhead)	Low	Medium (Russet Spotting)
Lettuce (Head/Iceberg)	Very Low	High (Russet Spotting)
Lime	Very Low	Medium (Mold Degreen)
Lychee	Medium	Medium (Accelerates Deterioration)
Mandarine	Very Low	Medium (Rind Breakdown, Decay)
Mango	Medium	High (Accelerates Ripening, Decay)
Mangosteen	Medium	High (Shorten Shelf life)
Mushrooms	Low	Medium
Nectarine	High	High (Decay)
Okra	Low	Medium (Increasing Pod Yellowing)
Olive	Low	Medium (Loss of Green Color and Flesh Firmness)
Onions	Very Low	Medium (Odor, Sprouting)
Orange (CA,AZ)	Very Low	Medium (Mold, Rind Breakdown)
Orange (FL,TX)	Very Low	Medium (Mold, Rind Breakdown)
Papaya	High	High (Accelerates Ripening, Decay)
Parsley	Very Low	High
Passion Fruit	Very High	High (Accelerates Ripening, Decay)
Peach	High	High (Decay)
Pear (Anjou,Bartlett/Bosc)	High	High (Decay)
Peas	Very Low	Medium (Accelerated Yellowing, Decay)
Pepper (Bell)	Low	Low (Accelerate Ripening, Color Change)
Pepper (Chile)	Low	Low (Accelerate Ripening, Color Change)
Persian Melon	Medium	High
Persimmon (Fuyu)	Low	High (Accelerates Softening, Decay)
Persimmon (Hachiya)	Low	High (Accelerates Softening, Decay)
Pineapple	Low	Low (Faster Degreening or Loss of Chlorophyll)
Pineapple (Guava)	Medium	Low (Faster Degreening or Loss of Chlorophyll)
Plantain	Low	High (Accelerates Ripening, Decay)
Plum/Prune	Medium	High (Decay)
Potato (Processing)	Very Low	Medium (Sprouting)
Potato (Seed)	Very Low	Medium
Potato (Table)	Very Low	Medium
Pumpkin	Low	Low
Quince	Low	High (Decay)
Radishes	Very Low	Low
Red Beet	Very Low	Low
Rambutan	High	High (Hastens Ripening, Undesirable color loss)
Sapota	Very High	High (Hastens Ripening)
Spinach	Very Low	High (Accelerates Yellowing)
Squash (Hard Skin)	Low	Low (Accelerates Yellowing, Stem Abscission)
Squash (Soft Skin)	Low	Medium (Accelerates Yellowing, Stem Abscission)
Squash (Summer)	Low	Medium (Accelerates Yellowing, Stem Abscission)
Sweet Potato	Very Low	Low
Tamarillo	Low	Medium (Undesirable Color Change)
Tangerine	Very Low	Medium (Rind Breakdown, Decay)
Tomato (Mature/Green)	Very Low	High (Shrink, Decay)
Tomato (Brkr/Lt Pink)	Medium	High (Shrink, Decay)
Tree-Tomato	High	Medium
Turnip (Greens)	Very Low	High
Watercress	Very Low	High
Watermelon	Low	High (Lose firmness)

Sources: Fresh Produce Manual for 1997 and the Sea Land Guide for Perishables

References

[1] BMC Public Health 2014, http://www.biomedcentral.com/1471-2458/14/143
http://www.nhlbi.nih.gov/health/health-topics/topics/obe/risks
[2] http://www.ncbi.nlm.nih.gov/pubmed/26024397
[3] http://www.cnpp.usda.gov/sites/default/files/dietary_guidelines_for_americans/PolicyDoc.pdf
[4] Fuhrman, Joel, The End of Dieting: How to live for life, New York, NY: HarperOne, an Imprint of HarperCollins Publishers, [2014] First edition.
http://www.diseaseproof.com/archives/healthy-food-eat-for-health-a-nutritarian-is-different-than-a-vegetarian.html
[5] Blatner, Dawn Jackson, The Flexitarian Diet: The Mostly Vegetarian Way to Lose Weight, Be Healthier, Prevent Disease, and Add Years to Your Life, McGraw-Hill, 2008.
[6] Delormier,T, K L Frohlich, and L Potvin, "Food and eating as social practice--understanding eating patterns as social phenomena and implications for public health," Sociology of Health and Illness, March 2009; 31(2): 215-28.
http://www.ncbi.nlm.nih.gov/pubmed/19220802
[7] http://www.vegetariantimes.com/article/vegetarianism-in-america/
[8] http://www.ncbi.nlm.nih.gov/pubmed/26024397
[9] Fuhrman, The End of Dieting: How to Live for Life.
[10] http://www.washingtonpost.com/blogs/wonkblog/wp/2014/06/17/the-generational-battle-of-butter-vs-margarine/
http://www.washingtonpost.com/news/wonkblog/wp/2015/08/07/the-butter-industry-probably-regrets-paying-for-this-study-that-shows-butter-is-bad-for-you/
[11] http://www.hsph.harvard.edu/nutritionsource/fiber-and-colon-cancer/
[12] http://www.ncbi.nlm.nih.gov/pmc/articles/PMC3435786/
[13] http://annals.org/article.aspx?articleid=1846638 http://news.sciencemag.org/health/2014/03/scientists-fix-errors-controversial-paper-about-saturated-fats
[14] Voodoo statistics and trust me science at http://www.pcf.org/atf/cf/%7B7c77d6a2-5859-4d60-af47-132fd0f85892%7D/Young,%20Stan-ABSTRACT.PDF
[15] http://www.washingtonpost.com/news/wonkblog/wp/2015/08/10/the-science-of-skipping-breakfast-how-government-nutritionists-may-have-gotten-it-wrong/http://advances.nutrition.org/content/5/1/7.full
[16] http://www.ncbi.nlm.nih.gov/pmc/articles/PMC3798081/
[17] http://www.ncbi.nlm.nih.gov/pubmed/26421384
[18] http://andrewbrownphd.com/2013/09/breakfast-bias-and-obesity
[19] http://jama.jamanetwork.com/article.aspx?articleid=1555137
[20] Fuhrman, The End of Dieting: How to Live for Life, p. 40.
[21] http://www.npr.org/sections/health-shots/2013/01/02/168437030/research-a-little-extra-fat-may-help-you-live-longer
[22] Fuhrman, The End of Dieting: How to Live for Life, pp 41-42.
[23] http://www.hsph.harvard.edu/nutritionsource/research-study-types/#laboratory-and-animal-studies
[24] Once Again, Physicists Debunk Faster-Than-Light Neutrinos http://news.sciencemag.org/2012/06/once-again-physicists-debunk-faster-light-neutrinos
[25] Cold fusion: A case study for scientific behavior http://undsci.berkeley.edu/lessons/pdfs/cold_fusion.pdf
[26] http://www.npr.org/sections/health-shots/2015/06/09/413140503/costs-of-slipshod-research-methods-may-be-in-the-billions
[27] Patrick Mustain, "Science for Sale: Big Food's Influence on Top Nutrition Research Org," Scientific American, June 15, 2015
[28] http://www.washingtonpost.com/news/wonkblog/wp/2015/08/07/the-butter-industry-probably-regrets-paying-for-this-study-that-shows-butter-is-bad-for-you/
[29] http://www.newrepublic.com/article/121806/nutrition-gap-are-doctors-ready-think-outside-pillbox
[30] Kelly M. Adams, W. Scott Butsch, and Martin Kohlmeier, "The State of Nutrition Education at US Medical Schools," Journal of Biomedical Education, Article ID 357627, January 2015.
http://www.hindawi.com/journals/jbe/aa/357627/

[31] Philip J Tuso, et al., "Nutritional Update for Physicians: Plant-Based Diets," Permanente Journal. 2013 Spring; 17(2): 61–66. http://www.ncbi.nlm.nih.gov/pmc/articles/PMC3662288/
[32] Vetter, Marion, et al., "What Do Resident Physicians Know about Nutrition? An Evaluation of Attitudes, Self-Perceived Proficiency and Knowledge," Journal of the American College of Nutrition, April 2008; 27(2): 287–298.
[33] http://www.hsph.harvard.edu/nutritionsource/
[34] http://lpi.oregonstate.edu/
[35] http://www.mayoclinic.org/healthy-lifestyle/nutrition-and-healthy-eating/basics/nutrition-basics/hlv-20049477
[36] http://www.berkeleywellness.com/
[37] http://news.health.com/2014/04/28/statin-users-eating-more-bad-food-than-a-decade-ago-study-shows/
[38] http://www.consumer-health.com/services/AreStatinstheMagicBullet.php
[39] http://www.globalresearch.ca/the-obesity-vaccine/31880
http://economictimes.indiatimes.com/magazines/panache/bacteria-may-give-you-type-2-diabetes/articleshow/47514655.cms
[40] http://www.canadianliving.com/food/cooking_school/flexitarian_lifestyle_how_to_eat_less_meat.php
[41] http://healthyeating.sfgate.com/wont-vegans-eat-honey-2938.html
[42] Fuhrman, J. Eat to Live, The Amazing Nutrient Rich Program for Fast and Sustained Weight Loss, Kindle Edition
[43] http://www.health.harvard.edu/family_health_guide/four-small-lifestyle-changes-can-mean-an-extra-14-years
[44] http://www.pnas.org/content/112/3/E277.full
[45] https://www.karger.com/Article/Pdf/318958
[46] http://www.ncbi.nlm.nih.gov/pmc/articles/PMC2684040/
[47] http://www.nist.gov/nvl/upload/Measures_for_Progress-MP275-FULL.pdf
[48] http://onlinelibrary.wiley.com/doi/10.1111/j.1467-789X.2006.00270.x/full
[49] http://www.amepc.org/tgc/article/view/4304/5761
[50] Leslie Pray, Rapporteur, Food Forum, Food and Nutrition Board, Institute of Medicine, Relationships Among the Brain, the Digestive System, and Eating Behavior, Workshop Summary, The National Academies Press ISBN 978-0-309-36683-0 134 pages (2015)
[51] James O Hill, Holly R Wyatt, John C Peters, "The Importance of Energy Balance, European Endocrinology, 2013;9(2):111–5 DOI:10.17925/EE.2013.09.02.111
http://www.touchendocrinology.com/sites/www.touchendocrinology.com/files/euendo9249-53_0.pdf
http://www.mayoclinic.org/healthy-lifestyle/weight-loss/in-depth/metabolism/art-20046508
[52] Speakman J R, and C Selman, "Physical activity and resting metabolic rate," Proceedings of the Nutrition Society, August 2003; 62(3):621-34 http://www.ncbi.nlm.nih.gov/pubmed/14692598
[53] http://www.fasebj.org/content/27/9/3837.long
[54] http://www.niddk.nih.gov/health-information/health-topics/weight-control/body-weight-planner/Pages/bwp.aspx
[55] http://www.nih.gov/news/health/aug2011/niddk-25.htm
[56] Lambert Adolphe Jacques Quetelet, Sur l'homme et le développement de ses facultés, ou Essai de physique sociale, 2 volumes, 1835
[57] Keys A, Fidanza F, Karvonen M J, Kimura N, Taylor H L, "Indices of Relative Weight and Obesity," Journal of Chronic Diseases, July 1, 1972; 25(6): 329-43.
[58] http://www.cdc.gov/healthyweight/assessing/bmi/adult_bmi/
[59] Fuhrman, Joel, The End of Dieting, pp. 6-7.
[60] https://people.maths.ox.ac.uk/trefethen/bmi.html
http://www.nydailynews.com/life-style/health/new-bmi-formula-fatter-article-1.1244317
[61] http://www.medpagetoday.com/Endocrinology/Obesity/47465
[62] http://press.endocrine.org/doi/full/10.1210/edrv.21.6.0415
[63] http://journals.plos.org/plosone/article?id=10.1371/journal.pone.0112355
[64] http://www.nhlbi.nih.gov/health-pro/guidelines/current/obesity-guidelines/e_textbook/txgd/4142.htm
http://www.ncbi.nlm.nih.gov/pmc/articles/PMC3193782/
[65] http://www.nhlbi.nih.gov/health-pro/guidelines/current/obesity-guidelines/e_textbook/txgd/4112.htm
[66] http://www.ncbi.nlm.nih.gov/pmc/articles/PMC3063466/
[67] http://annals.org/article.aspx?articleid=2468805

[68] http://www.cdc.gov/healthyweight/assessing/
[69] http://uk.reuters.com/article/2015/11/09/us-health-bellyfat-idUKKCN0SY2O520151109
http://annals.org/article.aspx?articleid=2468805
[70] http://www.webmd.com/diet/body-fat-measurement
Dympna Gallagher, Steven B Heymsfield, Moonseong Heo, Susan A Jebb, Peter R Murgatroyd, and Yoichi Sakamoto, "Healthy percentage body fat ranges: an approach for developing guidelines based on body mass index," http://ajcn.nutrition.org/content/72/3/694.full
[71] http://www.acefitness.org/acefit/healthy-living-article/60/112/what-are-the-guidelines-for-percentage-of/
[72] http://weightology.net/weightologyweekly/?page_id=146
[73] http://www.ncbi.nlm.nih.gov/pubmed/21085903
Guerra R S, Amaral T F, Marques E, Mota J, Restivo M T, "Accuracy of Siri and Brozek equations in the percent body fat estimation in older adults," Journal of Nutrition, Health and Aging, Nov 2010; 14(9):744-8
[74] http://weightology.net/weightologyweekly/?page_id=162
[75] http://www.ncbi.nlm.nih.gov/pmc/articles/PMC2495082/
http://weightology.net/weightologyweekly/?page_id=232
[76] http://www.cosmedusa.com/hires/marketing_literature/product_news/Product_News_Multi_compartment_model_EN_print.pdf
[77] http://weightology.net/weightologyweekly/?page_id=250
[78] http://www.cosmedusa.com/hires/marketing_literature/product_news/Product_News_Multi_compartment_model_EN_print.pdf
[79] http://www.ncbi.nlm.nih.gov/pubmed/17508096
http://weightology.net/weightologyweekly/?page_id=260
[80] http://ajcn.nutrition.org/content/64/3/524S.long
[81] http://rodrigoborges.com/principal/pdf/forca_09.pdf
[82] http://ajcn.nutrition.org/content/64/3/524S.long
[83] http://www.mayoclinic.org/healthy-lifestyle/fitness/expert-answers/body-fat-analyzers/faq-20057944
[84] http://ajcn.nutrition.org/content/34/12/2839.long
[85] http://www.ncbi.nlm.nih.gov/pubmed/9972188
[86] http://www.nature.com/ejcn/journal/v64/n2/full/ejcn2009111a.html
[87] http://ajcn.nutrition.org/content/75/2/245.full
[88] Ignasius Radix A P Jati, Vellingiri Vadivel, Donatus Nohr, and Hans Konrad Biesalski, "Nutrient density score of typical Indonesian foods and dietary formulation using linear programming," Public Health Nutrition: 15(12), 2185–2192
http://www.ncbi.nlm.nih.gov/pubmed/?term=Public+Health+Nutrition%3B+Dec2012%2C+Vol.+15+Issue+12%2C+p2185-2192%2C+8p
André Briend, Nicole Darmon, Elaine Ferguson, Juergen G. Erhardt, "Linear programming: A mathematical tool for analyzing and optimizing children's diets during the complementary feeding period," Journal of Pediatric Gastroenterology and Nutrition 36:12–22 http://ajcn.nutrition.org/content/75/2/245.full
[89] http://www.nutrisurvey.de/lp/lp.htm
[90] http://docs.scipy.org/doc/scipy-0.15.1/reference/generated/scipy.optimize.linprog.html
[91] http://ajcn.nutrition.org/content/82/4/721.full
[92] http://www.drfuhrman.com/library/andi-food-scores.aspx
[93] http://www.ncbi.nlm.nih.gov/pubmed/16321593
[94] http://www.active.com/fitness/articles/dietdetective-com-energy-and-nutrient-density-explained
http://www.ncbi.nlm.nih.gov/pmc/articles/PMC4049200/
http://www.ncbi.nlm.nih.gov/pmc/articles/PMC4049200/#R10
http://www.cdc.gov/pcd/issues/2014/13_0390.htm
Di Noia J, "Defining Powerhouse Fruits and Vegetables: A Nutrient Density Approach," Preventing Chronic Disease 2014; 11:130390. DOI: http://dx.doi.org/10.5888/pcd11.130390
[95] http://www.thelancet.com/pdfs/journals/lancet/PIIS0140673608615317.pdf
[96] http://www.ncbi.nlm.nih.gov/pubmed/25012199
[97] http://www.acc.org/latest-in-cardiology/articles/2014/09/01/15/30/is-a-greater-amount-of-visceral-adiposity-associated-with-htn

[98] http://www.fda.gov/Food/IngredientsPackagingLabeling/LabelingNutrition/ucm063367.htm
[99] http://www.businessinsider.com/american-pizza-community-is-objecting-to-calorie-regulations-2015-6#ixzz3fUdevmYT
https://s3.amazonaws.com/public-inspection.federalregister.gov/2015-16865.pdf
[100] http://www.fda.gov/Food/GuidanceRegulation/GuidanceDocumentsRegulatoryInformation/LabelingNutrition/ucm064928.htm
[101] http://www.cornucopia.org/2015/06/close-the-loophole-allowing-conventional-cows-on-organic-farms/
[102] http://choosemyplate.gov/weight-management-calories/calories/empty-calories-amount.html
[103] http://www.fda.gov/Food/IngredientsPackagingLabeling/LabelingNutrition/ucm274593.htm
[104] http://www.fda.gov/Food/GuidanceRegulation/GuidanceDocumentsRegulatoryInformation/LabelingNutrition/ucm385663.htm
[105] http://online.wsj.com/public/resources/documents/print/WSJ_-A002-20150307.pdf
[106] Lin Yang, and Graham A Colditz, "Prevalence of Overweight and Obesity in the United States, 2007-2012," JAMA Internal Medicine. Published online June 22, 2015.
http://archinte.jamanetwork.com/article.aspx?articleid=2323411
http://www.washingtonpost.com/news/wonkblog/wp/2015/08/25/the-fda-is-making-a-big-change-to-nutrition-labels-and-its-probably-a-mistake/
[107] http://ajcn.nutrition.org/content/34/3/362.full.pdf+html
http://www.ncbi.nlm.nih.gov/pubmed/6259925
[108] https://hms.harvard.edu/sites/default/files/assets/Sites/Longwood_Seminars/Nutrition_3_5_13.pdf
[109] http://www.nature.com/articles/srep10041
[110] http://www.health.com/health/gallery/0,,20708150,00.html
[111] http://www.heart.org/HEARTORG/GettingHealthy/NutritionCenter/HealthyEating/Understanding-Food-Nutrition-Labels_UCM_300132_Article.jsp#.VibzrH6rTDc
[112] http://io9.com/what-if-natural-products-came-with-a-list-of-ingredient-1503320184
[113] http://www.ncbi.nlm.nih.gov/pmc/articles/PMC3736515/ http://ajcn.nutrition.org/content/99/5/1223S.long
[114] http://www.mayoclinic.org/diseases-conditions/high-blood-cholesterol/in-depth/trans-fat/art-20046114
[115] http://www.ncbi.nlm.nih.gov/pubmed/20071648
[116] http://www.health.harvard.edu/staying-healthy/the-truth-about-fats-bad-and-good
[117] http://health.gov/dietaryguidelines/2015-scientific-report/11-chapter-6/d6-2.asp
[118] http://www.hsph.harvard.edu/nutritionsource/carbohydrates/carbohydrates-and-blood-sugar/
[119] http://www.health.harvard.edu/healthy-eating/glycemic_index_and_glycemic_load_for_100_foods
[120] http://www.aicr.org/press/health-features/health-talk/2015/04-april/recommendations-red-meat-saturated-fat-1.html?referrer=https://www.google.com/
[121] http://www.iarc.fr/en/media-centre/pr/2015/pdfs/pr240_E.pdf
[122] http://www.fda.gov/Food/FoodborneIllnessContaminants/ChemicalContaminants/ucm053569.htm#1
http://www.ncbi.nlm.nih.gov/pubmed/12623671
[123] http://iom.nationalacademies.org/activities/nutrition/summarydris/~/media/files/activity%20files/nutrition/dris/uls%20for%20vitamins%20and%20elements.pdf
[124] http://lpi.oregonstate.edu/mic/vitamins/vitamin-A#food-sources
[125] http://livertox.nih.gov/Niacin.htm
http://lpi.oregonstate.edu/mic/vitamins/niacin
http://pennstatehershey.adam.com/content.aspx?productId=107&pid=33&gid=000335
[126] http://www.ncbi.nlm.nih.gov/pubmed/16320662
[127] https://www.drfuhrman.com/library/folic_acid_dangers_and_prenatal_vitamins.aspx
http://chriskresser.com/folate-vs-folic-acid/
http://lpi.oregonstate.edu/mic/vitamins/folate
[128] http://www.mayoclinic.org/healthy-lifestyle/nutrition-and-healthy-eating/expert-answers/vitamin-c/faq-20058030
[129] http://www.mayoclinic.org/healthy-lifestyle/nutrition-and-healthy-eating/expert-answers/vitamin-d-toxicity/faq-20058108
[130] http://lpi.oregonstate.edu/mic/vitamins/vitamin-E#reference72

http://www.ianrpubs.unl.edu/pages/publicationD.jsp?publicationId=295
[131] http://lpi.oregonstate.edu/mic/articles/vitamins/vitamin-k
[132] http://iom.nationalacademies.org/Activities/Nutrition/SummaryDRIs/~/media/Files/Activity%20Files/Nutrition/DRIs/ULs%20for%20Vitamins%20and%20Elements.pdf
[133] http://lpi.oregonstate.edu/mic/minerals/calcium#safety
http://www.nlm.nih.gov/medlineplus/ency/article/000332.htm
[134] http://lpi.oregonstate.edu/mic/minerals/iron#nutrient-interactions
[135] https://ods.od.nih.gov/factsheets/Iron-HealthProfessional/
http://www.nlm.nih.gov/medlineplus/ency/article/007478.htm
[136] https://ods.od.nih.gov/factsheets/Magnesium-HealthProfessional/\
http://lpi.oregonstate.edu/mic/minerals/magnesium#safety
[137] http://www.webmd.com/vitamins-and-supplements/nutrition-vitamins-11/fat-water-nutrient?page=4
[138] http://ajcn.nutrition.org/content/87/2/379.full
[139] https://ods.od.nih.gov/factsheets/Selenium-HealthProfessional/
[140] http://lpi.oregonstate.edu/mic/minerals/selenium#safety
[141] http://www.hsph.harvard.edu/nutritionsource/the-new-salt-controversy/
[142] http://lpi.oregonstate.edu/mic/minerals/sodium#toxicity
[143] http://www.nature.com/jhh/journal/v16/n4/full/1001374a.html
[144] http://www.hsph.harvard.edu/news/press-releases/processed-meats-unprocessed-heart-disease-diabetes/
[145] http://www.ncbi.nlm.nih.gov/pmc/articles/PMC3680013/
[146] http://jaha.ahajournals.org/content/4/8/e001959.full
[147] Masoud Amiri and Roya Kelishad, "Can Salt Hypothesis Explain the Trends of Mortality from Stroke and Stomach Cancer in Western Europe?" International Journal of Preventive Medicine, June 2012; 3(6): 377–378. http://www.ncbi.nlm.nih.gov/pmc/articles/PMC3389433/
[148] http://www.ncbi.nlm.nih.gov/pubmed/24114476
[149] https://ods.od.nih.gov/factsheets/Zinc-HealthProfessional/http://lpi.oregonstate.edu/mic/minerals/zinc
[150] http://www.dsld.nlm.nih.gov/dsld/.
[151] http://www.fda.gov/Food/IngredientsPackagingLabeling/FoodAdditivesIngredients/ucm094211.htm
[152] http://www.nrdc.org/food/files/safety-loophole-for-chemicals-in-food-report.pdf
http://foodbabe.com/2015/04/24/dangerous-ingredient/
[153] http://www.hsph.harvard.edu/nutritionsource/healthy-drinks/artificial-sweeteners/
http://www.nlm.nih.gov/medlineplus/ency/article/007492.htm
[154] http://www.fda.gov/Food/IngredientsPackagingLabeling/FoodAdditivesIngredients/ucm397725.htm#SummaryTable
[155] http://www.fda.gov/AboutFDA/Transparency/Basics/ucm214864.htm
[156] http://www.fda.gov/AboutFDA/Transparency/Basics/ucm214865.htm
[157] http://www.stevia.net/fda.htm
[158] http://www.fda.gov/ForConsumers/ConsumerUpdates/ucm048951.htm
http://www.ift.org/~/media/Food%20Technology/pdf/2009/04/0409feat_NewColor.pdf
[159] http://www.ift.org/~/media/Food%20Technology/pdf/2009/04/0409feat_NewColor.pdf
http://www.fda.gov/ForIndustry/ColorAdditives/RegulatoryProcessHistoricalPerspectives/
http://www.foodsafetynews.com/2010/07/popular-food-dyes-linked-to-cancer-adhd-and-allergies/#.VaVt_PlViko
[160] http://www.mayoclinic.org/diseases-conditions/adhd/expert-answers/adhd/faq-20058203
[161] http://ensia.com/features/banned-in-europe-safe-in-the-u-s/ http://www.onlineholistichealth.com/food-dyes-additives-proven-unsafe/#sthash.bpKOnqtG.dpuf http://www.shape.com/blogs/shape-your-life/13-banned-foods-still-allowed-us http://ensia.com/features/banned-in-europe-safe-in-the-u-s/
[162] http://ensia.com/features/banned-in-europe-safe-in-the-u-s/
[163] http://www.diagnose-me.com/treatment/BHT-butylated-hydroxytoluene.html
[164] http://ntp.niehs.nih.gov/ntp/roc/content/profiles/butylatedhydroxyanisole.pdf
Botterweck A A, Verhagen H, Goldbohm R A, Kleinjans J, van den Brandt P A., Intake of butylated hydroxyanisole and butylated hydroxytoluene and stomach cancer risk: results from analyses in the Netherlands Cohort Study, Food and Chemical Toxicology 38(7): 599-605.
[165] http://www.berkeleywellness.com/healthy-eating/food-safety/article/two-preservatives-avoid

[166] http://ajcn.nutrition.org/content/90/1/1.full
http://fyi.uwex.edu/meats/files/2012/02/Nitrate-and-nitrite-in-cured-meat_10-18-2012.pdf
[167] http://www.accessdata.fda.gov/scripts/cdrh/cfdocs/cfCFR/CFRSearch.cfm?fr=172.175
[168] http://fyi.uwex.edu/meats/files/2012/02/Nitrate-and-nitrite-in-cured-meat_10-18-2012.pdf
[169] http://www.ncbi.nlm.nih.gov/pubmed/22487433
[170] National Academy of Sciences, "The health effects of nitrate, nitrite and n-nitroso compounds," National Academy Press, Washington, DC, 1981.
[171] http://ajcn.nutrition.org/content/90/1/1.full
[172] http://www.accessdata.fda.gov/scripts/cdrh/cfdocs/cfCFR/CFRSearch.cfm?fr=172.170
[173] http://toxnet.nlm.nih.gov/cgi-bin/sis/search/a?dbs+hsdb:@term+@DOCNO+726
[174] http://ajcn.nutrition.org/content/90/1/11.full
[175] http://www.nejm.org/doi/full/10.1056/NEJMc062800
[176] http://www.ncbi.nlm.nih.gov/pmc/articles/PMC3545899/
.http://cardiovascres.oxfordjournals.org/content/89/3/492
http://www.feingold.org/Research/PDFstudies/Sebranek2007.pdf
[177] http://www.who.int/ipcs/publications/cicad/cicad26_rev_1.pdf
[178] http://www.ncbi.nlm.nih.gov/pubmed/25497115
[179] http://articles.latimes.com/2011/sep/08/news/la-heb-skinnygirl-margarita-sodium-benzoate-20110908
[180] http://www.fda.gov/Food/FoodborneIllnessContaminants/ChemicalContaminants/ucm055815.htm
http://www.fda.gov/Food/FoodborneIllnessContaminants/ChemicalContaminants/ucm055131.htm
[181] http://www.fda.gov/ICECI/ComplianceManuals/CompliancePolicyGuidanceManual/ucm074468.htm
[182] http://www.fda.gov/ForConsumers/ConsumerUpdates/ucm048613.htm
[183] http://www.sciencedaily.com/releases/2010/11/101103135352.htm
[184] http://ajcn.nutrition.org/content/78/3/579S.full
[185] http://ajcn.nutrition.org/content/78/3/579S.full
[186] http://www.ncbi.nlm.nih.gov/pubmed/17022438
[187] http://ajcn.nutrition.org/content/87/2/379.full
[188] http://www.medicalnewstoday.com/articles/284096.php#potential_health_risks_of_consuming_fennel\
[189] http://www.ncbi.nlm.nih.gov/pmc/articles/PMC3342754/
[190] http://www.ncbi.nlm.nih.gov/pubmed/26024397
[191] http://www.fda.gov/ForConsumers/ConsumerUpdates/ucm094536.htm
[192] http://www.fda.gov/Food/GuidanceRegulation/GuidanceDocumentsRegulatoryInformation/LabelingNutrition/ucm064916.htm
[193] http://choosemyplate.gov/healthy-eating-tips/tips-for-vegetarian.html
[194] https://ods.od.nih.gov/Health_Information/Dietary_Reference_Intakes.aspx
http://www.ncbi.nlm.nih.gov/books/NBK234926/
[195] http://www.hsph.harvard.edu/nutritionsource/fiber-and-colon-cancer/
[196] http://www.health.state.mn.us/divs/hpcd/chp/cdrr/nutrition/facts/wholegrains.html
[197] http://www.ncbi.nlm.nih.gov/pubmed/19878856
[198] http://www.nutrition-and-you.com/quinoa.html
[199] http://lpi.oregonstate.edu/mic/dietary-factors/phytochemicals/soy-isoflavones#food-sources
[200] http://www.ncbi.nlm.nih.gov/pubmed/15867311
[201] http://www.seriouseats.com/2014/06/shopping-cooking-guide-different-tofu-types.html
[202] http://www.ncbi.nlm.nih.gov/pubmed/2380647
[203] http://www.popsugar.com/fitness/Nutritional-Comparison-Tofu-Tempeh-Seitan-Recipes-18692390
[204] http://www.ncbi.nlm.nih.gov/pmc/articles/PMC3786657
Rizos, E C, et al., "Association between omega-3 fatty acid supplementation and risk of major cardiovascular disease events: a systematic review and meta-analysis," Journal of the American Medical Association, 308(10):1024–1033.
[205] http://jnci.oxfordjournals.org/content/early/2013/07/09/jnci.djt174.full
[206] http://link.springer.com/article/10.1007%2Fs10555-012-9369-5
[207] http://www.ncbi.nlm.nih.gov/pubmed/12737006

[208] http://www.nlm.nih.gov/medlineplus/ency/imagepages/19303.htm
[209] http://lpi.oregonstate.edu/mic/dietary-factors/phytochemicals/resveratrol)
[210] http://www.ncbi.nlm.nih.gov/pmc/articles/PMC4017674/
[211] http://www.sparkpeople.com/resource/nutrition_articles.asp?id=297
[212] European Journal of Nutrition, September 2012; 51(6): 637–663. http://www.ncbi.nlm.nih.gov/pmc/articles/PMC3419346/
[213] ws.yahoo.com/apple-day-may-not-keep-doctor-away-study-151026289.html http://www.ncbi.nlm.nih.gov/pmc/articles/PMC442131/
[214] http://www.ncbi.nlm.nih.gov/pmc/articles/PMC442131
[215] https://www.drfuhrman.com/library/andi-food-scores.aspx
[216] https://hms.harvard.edu/sites/default/files/assets/Sites/Longwood_Seminars/Nutrition_3_5_13.pdf
[217] http://www.hsph.harvard.edu/nutritionsource/pyramid-full-story/
[218] http://www.allergykids.com/what-you-can-do/nutrient-density-and-phytochemical-rich-foods/
[219] http://www.doctoroz.com/article/fuhrman-superfoods-g-bombs?page=1https://www.drfuhrman.com/library/foodpyramid.aspx
[220] http://www.med.umich.edu/umim/clinical/pyramid/index.htm http://www.med.umich.edu/opm/newspage/2005/pyramid.htm http://www.med.umich.edu/umim/food-pyramid/about.html
[221] http://www.med.umich.edu/umim/food-pyramid/fruits_and_vegetables.html
[222] Ray Kurzwell and Terry Grossman, Transcend: Nine Steps to Living Well Forever, Rodale Books, 2009, p 239.
[223] http://www.mayoclinic.org/healthy-lifestyle/nutrition-and-healthy-eating/multimedia/mayo-clinic-healthy-weight-pyramid/img-20008111 http://diet.mayoclinic.org/diet/eat/follow-the-mayo-clinic-healthy-weight-pyramid https://www.bcbsri.com/BCBSRIWeb/images/pdfs/fn14_hwp.pdf
[224] http://oldwayspt.org/sites/default/files/files/V&V_pyramid_flyer.pdf
[225] http://oldwayspt.org/resources/heritage-pyramids/mediterranean-pyramid/overview
[226] http://ajcn.nutrition.org/content/61/6/1402S.full.pdf
[227] http://www.vegetariannutrition.org/food-pyramid.pdf
[228] http://www.drweil.com/drw/u/ART02995/Dr-Weil-Anti-Inflammatory-Food-Pyramid.html
[229] http://www.eufic.org/article/en/expid/food-based-dietary-guidelines-in-europe/ http://www.huffingtonpost.com/food-republic/food-pyramids-around-the-world_b_874409.html
[230] http://www.ncbi.nlm.nih.gov/pmc/articles/PMC4013194/ http://www.ncbi.nlm.nih.gov/pubmed/25929408
[231] http://www.ncbi.nlm.nih.gov/pubmed/11794489
[232] Yoni Freedhoff, MD, Assistant Professor of Family Medicine, University of Ottawa http://health.usnews.com/health-news/blogs/eat-run/2012/11/28/of-course-theres-such-a-thing-as-a-bad-food
[233] https://patentimages.storage.googleapis.com/pages/US1205240-0.png
[234] Mark B McClellan, "Changing the American Diet," Speech before Harvard School of Public Health, July 1, 2003. http://www.fda.gov/newsevents/speeches/ucm053648.htm
[235] http://www.hsph.harvard.edu/nutritionsource/healthy-eating-plate-vs-usda-myplate/
[236] http://www.todaysdietitian.com/newarchives/070113p16.shtml
[237] http://www.howjsay.com/index.php?word=carrageenan&submit=Submit
[238] http://www.hsph.harvard.edu/nutritionsource/recipes-2/
[239] https://www.blueapron.com/
[240] https://www.hellofresh.com/
[241] https://www.plated.com/
[242] https://thepurplecarrot.com/
[243] http://www.personalchef.com/personal_chef_faqs.php#.VhO-8flViko
[244] http://personal.rhul.ac.uk/uhah/058/perfect_parking.pdf http://discovermagazine.com/2011/sep/18-your-brain-knows-lot-more-than-you-realize
[245] http://www.hsph.harvard.edu/nutritionsource/healthy-drinks/soft-drinks-and-disease/
[246] http://www.mayoclinic.org/healthy-lifestyle/nutrition-and-healthy-eating/in-depth/artificial-sweeteners/art-20046936?pg=1
[247] http://www.extension.umn.edu/food/food-safety/preserving/general/water-for-food-preservation/

[248] http://www.fda.gov/Food/GuidanceRegulation/FSMA/ucm304045.htm#prevention
[249] http://water.epa.gov/drink/hotline/
[250] http://www.health.state.mn.us/divs/eh/water/factsheet/com/bottledwater.html
[251] http://www.nrdc.org/thisgreenlife/0902.asp
[252] http://www.nrdc.org/water/drinking/bw/exesum.asp
[253] http://www.fda.gov/Food/GuidanceRegulation/FSMA/
[254] http://www.ncbi.nlm.nih.gov/pmc/articles/PMC1642697/
https://www.jstage.jst.go.jp/article/endocrj/57/5/57_K10E-077/_pdf
[255] http://www.thesimpledollar.com/dont-eat-out-as-often-188365/
[256] http://www.forbes.com/sites/halahtouryalai/2013/09/25/lunchtime-americans-spend-nearly-1k-annually-eating-out-for-lunch/
[257] http://www.webmd.com/food-recipes/buffet-bellyaches
[258] http://www.foodsafetynews.com/restaurant-inspections-in-your-area/#.VeXIHvlViko
http://www.nytimes.com/1999/08/25/dining/eating-well-salad-bars-how-clean-are-they.html
[259] http://www.nytimes.com/2013/04/07/magazine/yes-healthful-fast-food-is-possible-but-edible.html?pagewanted=all&_r=0
[260] http://www.dirtcandynyc.com/menus
[261] http://vedgerestaurant.com/
[262] http://www.cinnamonsnail.com/
[263] http://www.peta.org/living/food/best-vegan-food-trucks/
[264] http://www.berkeleywellness.com/healthy-eating/diet-weight-loss/nutrition/article/truth-about-detox-diets
[265] http://www.ncbi.nlm.nih.gov/pubmed/26375358
[266] http://www.ncbi.nlm.nih.gov/pmc/articles/PMC2988700/
[267] http://www.fasebj.org/content/29/1_Supplement/597.7
[268] http://www.ncbi.nlm.nih.gov/pmc/articles/PMC4268877/
[269] http://www.dalswildlifesite.com/rapaciousbirdsandowlsbio.htm
[270] http://www.ncbi.nlm.nih.gov/pmc/articles/PMC535701/
[271] http://ajcn.nutrition.org/content/85/2/426.full
[272] http://www.ncbi.nlm.nih.gov/pubmed/21641703/
[273] http://www.ncbi.nlm.nih.gov/pubmed/25127476
[274] Jamie Koufman and Jordan Stern, "Dropping Acid: The Reflux Diet Cookbook & Cure," The Reflux Cookbooks, LLC, p. 35.
[275] http://rspb.royalsocietypublishing.org/content/282/1809/20150229
[276] http://www.cookinglight.com/cooking-101/techniques/cooking-questions-tips/print?print=
[277] http://www.mayoclinic.org/diseases-conditions/diabetes/expert-answers/diabetes/faq-20057835
[278] http://www.health.harvard.edu/heart-health/chocolate-pros-and-cons-of-this-sweet-treat
[279] http://www.uchospitals.edu/online-library/content=P07872
[280] http://www.ncbi.nlm.nih.gov/pubmed/14692598
[281] http://www.nature.com/ijo/journal/v30/n4s/full/0803520a.html
[282] http://ajcn.nutrition.org/content/82/1/222S.long
http://www.uchospitals.edu/online-library/content=P07872
http://www.mayoclinic.org/healthy-lifestyle/weight-loss/expert-answers/weight-loss/faq-20058292
[283] http://strongertogether.coop/food-coops/food-co-op-impact-study/
http://www.foodcoopinitiative.coop/content/co-op-directories
[284] http://www.vrg.org/blog/2012/10/15/starting-a-vegan-food-manufacturing-company-using-a-co-packer/
http://www.governing.com/topics/urban/portland-has-worlds-first-vegan-mini-mall.html
http://thevegantruth.blogspot.com/2013/12/100-vegan-ownedvegan-businesses_15.html
http://www.onecommunityranch.org/food-production-infrastructure/
https://globalconnections.hsbc.com/us/en/articles/cdn-cheese-vegans-catches-south-border
http://businessfacilities.com/2012/08/vegan-manufacturing-facility-to-open-in-columbia-mo/
[285] http://www.health.harvard.edu/blog/panel-suggests-stop-warning-about-cholesterol-in-food-201502127713
[286] http://www.hsph.harvard.edu/nutritionsource/media/

[287] http://www.healthnewsreview.org/toolkit/tips-for-understanding-studies/does-the-language-fit-the-evidence-association-versus-causation/
[288] http://www.thehastingscenter.org/Publications/BriefingBook/Detail.aspx?id=2156#ixzz3m8mz18Sa
[289] http://www.ncbi.nlm.nih.gov/pmc/articles/PMC3293157/
[290] http://www.ncbi.nlm.nih.gov/pmc/articles/PMC4560115/
[291] BMJ 2015;351:h4183   http://www.bmj.com/content/351/bmj.h4183
[292] http://www.jmir.org/2015/8/e209/
[293] https://www.nlm.nih.gov/medlineplus/healthywebsurfing.html
http://www.cancer.gov/about-cancer/managing-care/using-trusted-resources
[294] https://www.nlm.nih.gov/services/guide.html
[295] http://advances.nutrition.org/content/5/1/7.full
[296] http://lpi.oregonstate.edu/mic/food-beverages/cruciferous-vegetables#disease-prevention
[297] http://www.ncbi.nlm.nih.gov/pmc/articles/PMC3074486/
[298] http://lpi.oregonstate.edu/mic/dietary-factors/phytochemicals/resveratrol
[299] http://www.ars.usda.gov/Services/docs.htm?docid=15866

www.ingramcontent.com/pod-product-compliance
Lightning Source LLC
Chambersburg PA
CBHW081358290426
44110CB00018B/2405